Alzheimer's Disease and Marriage

Sage Series in
Clinical Nursing Research

The purpose of the **Sage Series in Clinical Nursing Research**, is to provide a concise description of the research on specific issues in nursing that are relevant to the practitioner. Authors report their own research findings and examine other important research in that area, paying close attention to the implications for practice and specifically addressing intervention techniques. The series will inform the nurse researcher of some of the significant research being conducted and help practicing nurses enhance their expertise.

In this series . . .

Alzheimer's Disease and Marriage

An Intimate Account

Lore K. Wright

Sage Series in Clinical Nursing Research

SAGE Publications
International Educational and Professional Publisher
Newbury Park   London   New Delhi

For information address:

SAGE Publications, Inc.
2455 Teller Road
Newbury Park, California 91320

SAGE Publications Ltd.
6 Bonhill Street
London EC2A 4PU
United Kingdom

SAGE Publications India Pvt. Ltd.
M-32 Market
Greater Kailash I
New Delhi 110 048 India

Printed in the United States of America

Library of Congress Cataloging-in-Publication Data

Wright, Lore K.
   Alzheimer's disease and marriage / Lore K. Wright.
      p.   cm.—(Clinical nursing research)
   Includes bibliographical references and index.
   ISBN 0-8039-4521-3 (cl).—ISBN 0-8039-4522-1 (pb)
   1. Alzheimer's disease—Patients—Family relationships.
2. Marriage—Psychological aspects. I. Title. II. Series:
Clinical nursing research (Unnumbered)
   [DNLM: 1. Alzheimer's Disease—psychology. 2. Marriage—
psychology. WM 220 W951a]
RC523.W75 1993
155.6'45—dc20
DNLM/DLC   92-48987

93 94 95 96 10 9 8 7 6 5 4 3 2 1

Sage Production Editor: Diane S. Foster

To Victor: The best is yet to be. . . .

Contents

Foreword

This book is about profound love and profound loss. Older spouse caregivers of persons with probable Alzheimer's disease experience the final years of their marriages in long anticipatory bereavement. Their loved ones can still sense affection, but slowly and deliberately the disease erases their ability to remember and to problem solve and, perhaps most tragically, to know one's self.

What is the impact of this progressive deterioration in one spouse on the marital relationship? To date, caregiving research sheds only dim light on this question due to the task of tracing out patterns of impact, response, and ultimate influence. Only by peering deeply into marriages and by obtaining highly personal data on individual behavior can such an analysis be accomplished. This is precisely what Lore Wright has done in this book—taken us behind closed doors for "an intimate account."

Most readers will approach this research with the widely accepted knowledge that providing for a demented spouse is challenging and highly stressful. However, all will finish it with new awareness of the manner in which dementia invades various dimensions of marriage and corrodes patterns of interaction and how older spouses respond to such transformations. The contrasting experiences of healthy older couples, presented simultaneously, bring the impact of Alzheimer's disease and its meaning for human development even more sharply into focus. As such, this story unfolds with important messages for gerontologists, geriatric nurses, and caregivers whose spouses are victims of cognitive impairment. Gerontologists will appreciate the linked-sample methodology, which breaks new ground in caregiving research by assigning value to reports from afflicted spouses. Gerontologists also will appreciate the theoretical discussions grappling with the question, When does human development cease in a cognitively impaired person? Nurses will find answers to vexing clinical questions related to caring for the caregiver. And, perhaps most importantly, caregivers will discover unique approaches to managing the personal and interpersonal changes they are experiencing as a result of their spouses' affliction.

This book represents the product of more than 3 years of painstaking research effort, coming to fruition in Lore Wright's postdoctoral fellowship at Duke University's Center for the Study of Aging and Human Development. It has been very rewarding for me, as one of her fellowship preceptors and nursing colleagues, to follow its careful development. I believe that readers who look through the window that has been carved so creatively into the private lives of these elderly couples will be similarly rewarded.

ELIZABETH COLERICK CLIPP

Acknowledgments

This study was partially supported by grants from the National Center for Nursing Research at NIH (1 F31 NRO 601-01 SRC), the Medical College of Georgia Research Institute (11-16-05-4220-66), and the National Institute on Aging (AG00029).

I also wish to acknowledge my mentors and colleagues who have contributed their intellectual support. In particular I wish to acknowledge James Dowd, my major professor, and Lennie Poon, Peter Martin, Linda Grant, Mary Conway, Sarah Gueldner, Elizabeth Colerick Clipp, and Linda George. Their interest and guidance helped shape and crystallize the ideas expressed in this work. I owe them gratitude—which cannot be repaid.

My gratitude also extends to the couples who shared their innermost thoughts with me. Without them this book could not have been written. It is their story that gives depth and meaning to this book. Their names and other distinguishing characteristics have been changed to protect the privacy of each spouse, but their courage will be apparent in the pages that follow. It is hoped that their courage can help others.

LORE K. WRIGHT

ONE

Overview

PURPOSE

The purpose of this book is to provide clinicians, researchers, students, and caregivers with in-depth knowledge about the impact of Alzheimer's disease on the marital relationship. The goal is to provide assessment strategies and intervention guidelines for situations where caregiver and afflicted spouse reside together in the community. The importance of such knowledge is underscored by the fact that more than 70% of all Alzheimer's disease afflicted persons are cared for in their homes and that one third to one half of all caregivers are spouses (Office of Technology Assessment [OTA], 1987, 1990).

This book goes beyond describing global marital happiness; instead, specific dimensions of the marital relationship such as household responsibilities, tension, companionship, affection and sexuality, and commitment are explored. Knowing how couples experience these issues and how they try to cope with problems in these areas can guide clinicians with interventions. For example, by knowing how couples view commitment to each other and their relationship, an appreciation for realistic plans for the future is gained. By knowing that high sexual activity can occur in afflicted spouses, specific assessment questions can be

1

posed. Health consequences of such situations, including emotional distress and bladder infections, can be addressed through counseling, teaching, and appropriate referrals. Such strategies can decrease the risk of aggravated health problems in caregivers, as well as decrease anger and hostility in afflicted spouses.

A DIFFERENT APPROACH

It is important to note that most other related studies provide information about caregivers only. In this book, however, the perspective of both the caregiver and the afflicted spouse, as well as the perspective of wives and husbands from a group of relatively healthy older couples, will be presented. The comparative approach with two groups of couples was chosen to bring the impact of Alzheimer's disease more clearly into focus and to differentiate illness impact from problems associated with aging in general.

Noelker and Kercher (1991) noted that the perspective of care receivers is one of the most neglected areas in gerontology. One reason for this neglect is that obtaining such information is a difficult task. Responses from afflicted spouses in this study were often tangential and required patience during the interview process. However, their answers—at least for some aspects of their marital relationship—showed surprisingly more awareness than might be expected. This book thus contributes to knowledge about the perceptions of a neglected population—those who receive care. Findings can help sensitize clinicians and researchers to the special problems faced by couples in the presence of Alzheimer's disease.

This book also contributes to understanding illness impact from a human developmental perspective. Although the disease itself and its debilitating effects are fully acknowledged and described, interpretations of these effects take people's past and present relationships and the anticipated future into consideration. The question whether Alzheimer's disease afflicted persons reach a point when human development ceases will also be addressed.

ALZHEIMER'S DISEASE: BIOLOGICAL, CLINICAL, AND SOCIAL PERSPECTIVE

Biological Aspects of Alzheimer's Disease

Alzheimer's disease is a progressively dementing disease. It is named after a German neurologist, Alois Alzheimer, who in 1907 described its characteristics. Microscopically, structural changes in the brain occur in the form of neurofibrillary tangles (hairlike structures wrapped around each other) and neuritic plaques (spherical structures composed of a protein called *amyloid*). Although structural changes in the brain are also found in older persons without dementia, it is the density of plaques and tangles that distinguishes Alzheimer's disease from normal aging (Cohen & Eisdorfer, 1986).

The structural changes in the brain's cortex affect what is referred to as higher brain functions: thinking, judgment, reasoning, speech, and language. In addition, structural changes in the hippocampus and other parts of the limbic system (which lie deep below the cerebral cortex) disrupt attention and memory and also may account for changes in emotional control and in personality that occur in Alzheimer's disease afflicted persons (Burns & Buckwalter, 1988; Cohen & Eisdorfer, 1986; Reisberg, 1983).

Even though the disease is fairly well defined microscopically, there is as yet no known cause, no single test to diagnose the illness definitively prior to autopsy, and no known cure. Intense biomedical research currently focuses on beta amyloid protein deposits that form the neuritic plaques. Joachim and Selkoe concluded that it seems likely "most, if not all, senile plaques contain beta amyloid protein deposits" (Joachim & Selkoe, 1989, p. B80). However, how beta amyloid is deposited in the brain and whether, once there, it becomes the primary cause of the structural changes associated with Alzheimer's disease or whether beta amyloid accumulates secondarily to some as yet unknown process remain unanswered questions (Joachim & Selkoe, 1989).

Clinical Aspects of Alzheimer's Disease

The illness tends to progress at an uneven rate and may span 8 to 25 years from symptom onset to death (OTA, 1987). Despite individual variation in symptom progression, several stages have been discerned. At the most global level, three stages occur. The first stage is marked by onset of memory loss, particularly for recent events. The second stage is marked by problems in language, motor ability, and recognition of objects. The third or terminal stage is marked by profound dementia with loss of continence, loss of ability to walk, and nearly complete loss of language (Sjogren, Sjogren, & Lundgren, 1952).

More detailed clinical phases have been identified and summarized by Reisberg (1983) with the Global Deterioration Scale (GDS), which lists seven stages and corresponding phases. Stage one is considered to be normal, with no cognitive decline. Stage two evidences very mild cognitive decline and is characterized by forgetfulness, but no objective deficits in social functioning are noticed. Stage three, the early confusional phase, is characterized by getting lost in unfamiliar places, co-workers becoming aware of poor performance, forgetting names, and misplacing objects; mild to moderate anxiety tends to be present. Stage four, the late confusional phase, is characterized by decreased knowledge of current and recent events, decreased concentration, decreased ability to travel and to handle finances, flattening of affect, and withdrawal from challenging situations. Denial is a common defense mechanism at this time. In stage five, the early dementia phase, the afflicted person can no longer survive without some assistance; some disorientation to time or place occurs, and the person may be unable to name close members of the family. Eating and toileting are still performed independently, but assistance with choosing proper clothing may be required. In stage six, the middle dementia phase, afflicted persons still know their own name but occasionally may forget the name of their spouse, on whom they are entirely dependent for survival. Knowledge of their past lives is sketchy, they require travel assistance, they may become incontinent, and personality and emotional changes begin to occur. Stage seven, the final or late dementia phase, is characterized by loss of all verbal abilities; the afflicted person is unable to walk, is incontinent of urine, and requires assistance with toileting and feeding.

The Global Deterioration Scale correlates significantly with other psychometric measurements and with computerized tomography scans and metabolic changes in Alzheimer's patients and is thus a useful clinical tool (Ferris et al., 1980; Reisberg, 1983). Another scale commonly used to evaluate cognitive performance is the Mini-Mental State exam, which assesses orientation, registration, attention and calculation, recall, and language (Folstein, Folstein, & McHugh, 1975). The maximum obtainable score is 30; a score of 24 or below is considered to be an indication of cognitive impairment. Respondents above age 60 who have an educational level of less than 8 years, however, should be given a cutoff point of 22 or 21 to consider a diagnosis of dementia (Anthony, LeResche, Niaz, von Korff, & Folstein, 1982; Magaziner, Bassett, & Hebel, 1987).

Social Aspects of Alzheimer's Disease

The onset of Alzheimer's disease is age related. Most commonly, the illness occurs after age 65, and 5%-7% of older people are said to be afflicted. It is misleading to quote a prevalence rate for all people over age 65, however, because higher rates occur with advancing age. Based on new findings reported by Evans et al. (1989), the prevalence rate is 10.3% between ages 65 and 74; it rises to 18.7% between ages 75 and 84; and above age 85 the rate is 47.2%.

These percentages translate into many cases. The number of severely demented persons in the United States is quoted often as 1.5 million, and an additional 1 to 5 million persons are reported to have mild to moderate mental impairment (OTA, 1987). Projections indicate that unless cures or interventions for stabilizing the disease process of Alzheimer's disease are found, 7.4 million Americans will be afflicted by the year 2040 (OTA, 1987). But this may be an underestimation of cases; according to recent reports, as many as 11 to 13 million will be afflicted in the next century (Evans et al., 1989).

Clearly, with the aging of the American population and similar aging trends in most other developed countries, Alzheimer's disease is a major health concern. Although at present more than 70% of all afflicted persons are cared for in their homes and mostly by women (OTA, 1990; Stone, Cafferata, & Sangle, 1987), it is not known whether this pattern will continue, considering changes in family structure and different roles of women in contemporary society. Bergman and Cooper (1986) estimated that a decrease of only 5% in in-home care will result in more than doubling the demand for institutional places; this demand would lead to a breakdown in geriatric care and at the same time a decline in the quality of care for other patient groups.

To date, the presence of a spouse has been found to be the most important factor in preventing institutionalization (Colerick & George, 1986; Enright, 1991; Green & Monahan, 1987; Hamel et al., 1990; Lieberman & Kramer, 1991; Lund, Pett, & Caserta, 1987; Macken, 1986). Yet only sparse knowledge about the impact of Alzheimer's disease on the marital relationship is available. It is hoped that this book will increase our knowledge and understanding.

HUMAN DEVELOPMENT

A marital relationship implies that two people, a couple, interact with each other and with their environment over the course of a shared life. A couple's experiences will include happiness and contentment but also times of difficulties and distress. When the distress is Alzheimer's disease in one spouse, the couple's interactions will undergo change, but for both afflicted and caregiver spouse, the long-term marital relationship is the most important context for continuing interactions. This context has implications for human development.

It is argued that human development occurs throughout the life span and that interactions between people and the larger sociocultural environment are essential for development. But in addition, it is the presence of—or rather because of—life difficulties or crises that adult development occurs (Lerner, 1985; Riegel, 1973, 1976, 1979; Wright, 1989, 1991). Riegel (1976, 1979) termed such difficulties *asynchronies,* or the experience of asynchronized life dimensions between inner biological, individual psychological, and cultural, sociological aspects of life. It is only when we experience asynchronies, Riegel argues, that development can occur. Furthermore, outcomes of asynchronized life dimensions are not predetermined according to a person's "stage" in the life cycle; rather, as illness, conflicts, or environmental demands act on us, we, in turn, act and influence and change our environment in a never-ending dialectical exchange (Dowd, 1990; Georgoudi, 1983; Riegel, 1976, 1979). Thus, although an overall progression through the biological life span is acknowledged, greater emphasis is given to environmental influences and human initiative.

When applying a dialectical theory of human development to the marital relationship, the following assumptions are taken into consideration: (a) Couples have a shared history that has shaped the emotional and instrumental roles that partners carry out toward each other, and (b) their present relationship forms the basis of expectations for future emotional and instrumental caring. Such expectations, in turn, influence the present. Past, present, and future are intertwined (Ryff, 1984), or represent what Lehr (1982) has termed the *crossing point* (*Kreuzpunkt*) of existence. Whatever new life stressors or burdens (asynchronies) may occur, marital partners will incorporate their past dialectic history into their present relationship. This assimilation, together with anticipation of the future, leads to new developmental outcomes.

When we think of relatively healthy older couples, we have an image of supportive togetherness, idealized in Robert Browning's poem "Rabbi Ben Ezra": "Grow old along with me! / The best is yet to be, / The last of life, for which the first was made." But when one spouse has Alzheimer's disease, Robert Browning's poetic phrases seem like a broken promise. And yet these couples' interactions have a tenaciousness different from those that other family caregivers have with afflicted persons. Studies have shown

TABLE 1.1 Positive and Negative Outcomes With Asynchronized
Life Dimensions

Life Dimensions	Inner-Biological	Individual-Psychological
Individual-Psychological:	Control versus disorder	Concordance versus discordance
Cultural-Sociological:	Adaptation versus distortion	Acculturation versus exploitation

SOURCE: Adapted from *Foundations of Dialectical Psychology* (p. 9) by K. F. Riegel, 1979, New York: Academic Press.

that spouse caregivers spend more time in caregiving (Caserta, Lund, Wright, & Redburn, 1987), care for more severely impaired persons (Soldo & Myllyluoma, 1983), and "are the last to relinquish care [of a mate] to professionals" (Colerick & George, 1986, p. 496). Cantor (1983) concluded that the closer the kinship bond, the greater the amount of strain. These findings have raised concerns that the emotional and physical health of spouse caregivers will be adversely affected (Colerick & George, 1986; Eisdorfer, 1991). But can such caring by spouses in long-term relationships also be developmental? Could they evidence not only negative consequences but also positive developmental outcomes? And are all interactions and outcomes for caregiver-afflicted spouse dyads different from couples without cognitive impairment in one partner?

Outcomes are not predetermined, Riegel (1976, 1979) stated. Positive and negative changes can occur, depending on the type of actions taken while interacting with the immediate and larger environment. Table 1.1 categorizes positive and negative developmental outcomes that result from asynchronized biological, psychological, and cultural-sociological life dimensions. Outcomes are incorporated in the overall conceptual model presented in Figure 1.1; the model is intended to make explicit the theoretical assumptions argued thus far.

In the model, Alzheimer's disease is shown as a developmental asynchrony, impacting on the present marital relationship, which is intertwined with the spouses' shared past and anticipated future (Lehr, 1982; Ryff, 1984). Actions taken by spouses

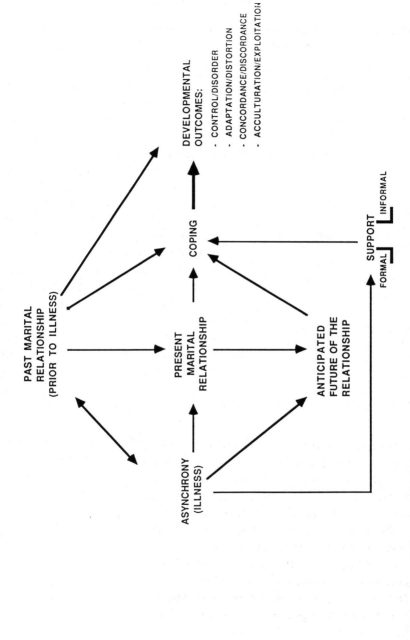

Figure 1.1. Overall Conceptual Model

9

are represented by coping, mediated by social support, which is obtained from the sociocultural environment. Together these variables lead to new developmental outcomes. Control or disorder, adaptation or distortion, concordance or discordance, acculturation or exploitation are examples of positive or negative outcomes (Riegel, 1976, 1979; Wright, 1989).

When stating that Alzheimer's disease is a developmental asynchrony and theoretically can lead to positive or negative outcomes, the afflicted spouses' progressively dementing, irreversible illness has to be acknowledged. The disease, simply put, affects the mind. But it is precisely mental capacity for shared meaning, thinking, and self-consciousness as part of a "mind" that is the essence of human interactions (Mead, 1977). *Mind*, according to Mead, is the capacity "to take the attitude of the other" or to have shared meaning in social interactions (Mead, 1977, p. 34). The mind orders perceptual experiences about others and the environment to give them meaning, or, in the words of W. I. Thomas (1923), experiences are ordered through the "prism of the mind." This ordering, in turn, leads to a "definition of the situation" (c.f. Coser, 1977, p. 521).

The "definition of the situation" and "taking the attitude of the other" are two guiding concepts in this work. Chappell and Orbach (1986) suggested that persons who are not able to form shared perspectives with other key persons (who cannot order experiences to give them similar meaning) may become defined as irrational or "senile." Only a rational or nonsenile person can interact in meaningful conduct with others because "rationality" implies that "the individual can take the attitude of the others, can control his actions by these attitudes, and control their actions through his own" (Mead, 1934, p. 334). By using this perspective of rationality, the extent to which the capacity for taking the attitude of the other is affected by illness and the extent to which the presence of illness becomes the prism for meaning in the couples' interactions versus relatively healthy couples can be assessed.

TABLE 1.2 Demographic Profile of AD and Well Group Couples

	AD group (n = 30 couples)	Well group (n = 17 couples)
Mean age	67.5	70
Range (age)	51-83	53-89
Mean years of education	13.3	14.1
Range (education)	4-22	8-22
Mean income per month	$1,862	$2,073
Range (income)	$580-$4,500	$1,200-$3,500
Mean years of marriage	38.1	44.6*
Range (marriage)	6-57	10-62

SOURCE: Adapted from "The Impact of Alzheimer's Disease on the Marital Relationship" by L. K. Wright, 1991, *The Gerontologist, 31*(2), p. 225. Copyright © The Gerontological Society of America. Used with permission.
NOTE: *$p < .002$.

CHARACTERISTICS OF
AD AND WELL COUPLES IN THIS STUDY

This book is based primarily on in-depth interviews with two groups of couples. One group consisted of 30 couples in which one spouse was in the early to middle stage of Alzheimer's disease and the other spouse functioned as the primary caregiver (hence referred to as the AD group). The other group consisted of 17 couples in which both spouses were relatively healthy—that is, neither spouse was cognitively impaired (hence referred to as the comparison or well group)—although common medical problems such as arthritis or heart disease were present. All couples resided in the community and were interviewed in their homes. Two couples were black; all others were white. A demographic profile of each group is presented in Table 1.2.

The AD and the well groups were similar in age, education, and monthly income. The AD group had more second and third marriages, however, resulting in an average length of marriage of 38 years for the AD group and 45 years for the well group. This difference is statistically significant. It is not known whether long-term happily married couples were more likely to agree to serving as comparison group subjects or whether the greater number of remarriages in the AD group is an indication of subtle

TABLE 1.3 Characteristics of Afflicted Spouses

	Male afflicted (n = 24)	Female afflicted (n = 6)
Mean age	68.7	70.2
Range (age)	56-82	59-83
Mean years of education	13.9	10.8*
Range (education)	6-22	9-12
Mean Mini-Mental State	17.8	18.7
Range (Mini-Mental)	8-28	10-24
Mean Global Deterioration Scale (GDS)	4.5	4
Range (GDS)	2-6	3-5

SOURCE: Adapted from "The Impact of Alzheimer's Disease on the Marital Relationship" by L. K. Wright, 1991, *The Gerontologist, 31*(2), p. 225. Copyright © The Gerontological Society of America. Used with permission.
NOTE: *$p < .01$.

early symptoms, experienced by afflicted spouses, that lead to relationship problems.

The AD group contained 24 male but only 6 female afflicted spouses. This ratio of 4:1 female to male caregivers is consistent with national trends for community caregivers (Stone et al., 1987). Age of the male and female afflicted spouses was similar, but mean years of eduction was significantly higher for the males (14 versus 11 years). They had been experiencing symptoms ranging from 1 to 11 years, with a mean of 5 years. All had a physician-established diagnosis of probable Alzheimer's disease. Assessment data obtained at the time of the interview indicated that they were in the early to middle stages of the disease: The mean Mini-Mental State score (Folstein et al., 1975) was 18, and the mean Global Deterioration Scale score (Reisberg, 1983) was 4.4. All still recognized their spouses by name and were able to communicate verbally. A profile of the afflicted spouses is presented in Table 1.3.

ORGANIZATION OF THE BOOK

This book is organized around five major dimensions of the marital relationship: (a) instrumental responsibilities, or simply household tasks, (b) tension, (c) companionship, (d) affection and sexuality, and (e) commitment. The marital relationship dimensions are based on Spanier and Thompson's (1982) Dyadic Marital Adjustment Rating Scale and additional questions pertinent to each dimension. The spouses' reported coping behaviors, as they relate to specific dimensions of the marital relationship, also will be presented. Spouses had answered the following questions to assess coping: "Do you have problems with . . . ?" "What specifically do you do when . . . ?" "Is there someone you can ask for help when . . . ?" It should be noted that although many of the spouses' answers are directly quoted in this book, the couples' names and other distinguishing characteristics have been changed to protect the privacy of each spouse.

In addition to the qualitative approach of assessing coping, each spouse's coping also was assessed quantitatively with the Jalowiec Coping Scale and its three subscales: confrontive or action-oriented coping; palliative or cognitive, stress-reducing coping; and emotive or negative emotional discharge coping (Jalowiec, 1988). Coping strategies based on Jalowiec's scale are presented in Chapter 7, while coping strategies based on qualitative data are discussed with each dimension of the marital relationship. Throughout the book other research reports will be included to support or question the findings from this study. Clinicians, researchers, and students interested in methodological and analysis issues are referred to the Appendix.

TWO

Household Tasks and Marriage

INTRODUCTION

In every marriage the performance of a number of instrumental or household tasks is required. These include the handling of family finances; the provision of nourishment, which requires grocery shopping and cooking; and the performance of maintenance tasks, such as cleaning house and making repairs. How these tasks are performed affects both spouses. Disagreement over tasks and the possibility of conflict are ever present.

EXPLORING HOUSEHOLD TASKS AND RESPONSIBILITIES

Household tasks that commonly occur as part of the marriage relationship were explored with three major questions: (a) Who does what, and who is responsible for what tasks? (b) How much agreement over tasks do both groups of couples report, and are husbands and wives similar or different in their assessment of agreement? and (c) What problems arise over money management, and how do couples cope with money management?

Who Does What?

Wives and husbands were asked "Who does what?" concerning a number of common household tasks and "Who takes the major responsibility to make sure these jobs get done?" Response options ranged from *I do it all the time* (5) to *I never or almost never do it* (1), adapted from the work by Emmons, Biernat, Tiedje, Lang, and Wortman (1990), who used similar questions with a different sample. The questions were asked with both spouses present. Cue cards listing the response options in large, bold print were used to help afflicted spouses with choosing their answers.

As shown in Figure 2.1, caregiver spouses performed and carried responsibility for all household tasks significantly more often than the afflicted spouses. Interesting is the less pronounced difference concerning "repairs," probably reflecting the greater number of male afflicted spouses in this study (24 males, 6 females) and hence some remaining gender role activity even in the presence of illness. The task of grocery shopping was a joint activity for many Alzheimer's couples; however, this activity represented more an outing for the afflicted spouse than the performance of a task. The choosing of groceries and the responsibility for planning the purchase of needed items clearly rested with the caregiver spouse.

A different pattern of performance and responsibility for household tasks was reported by the well couples. As shown in Figure 2.2, money management and responsibility for money were shared; that is, no significant differences between husbands and wives for this task were found. The other tasks, however, were divided along gender roles: Grocery shopping, cooking, and cleaning were significantly more often carried out by the wives, while repairs were significantly more often the domain of husbands. In a few instances, however, a wife answered, "I'm the electrician" or "He is the better cook," and on one occasion both responded simultaneously, "What cleaning?" and broke up in laughter. These cases are indicative of sociocultural changes, of greater flexibility in gender roles, even in this age group.

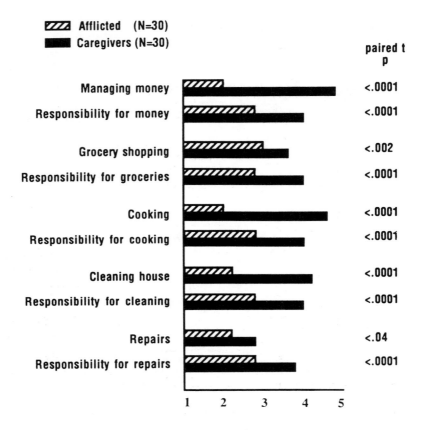

Figure 2.1. Performance of and Responsibility for Household Tasks: Mean Scores Reported by AD Group Couples

SOURCE: From "The Impact of Alzheimer's Disease on the Marital Relationship" by L. K. Wright, 1991, *The Gerontologist, 31*(2), p. 227. Copyright © The Gerontological Society of America. Reprinted with permission.

Agreement Over Tasks

Because there is such obvious difference in the quantity of household tasks performed by husbands and wives of the two groups, did one group also experience higher disagreements over these matters? Agreement or consensus was assessed with one of the subscales of Spanier and Thompson's (1982) Dyadic

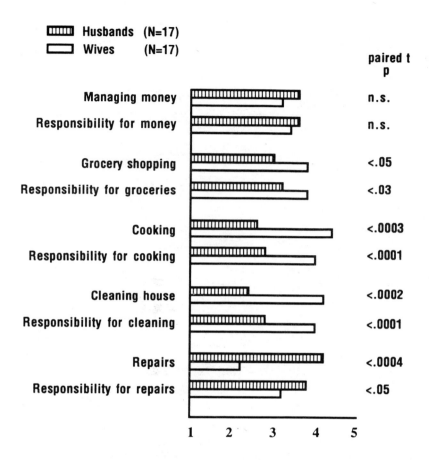

Figure 2.2. Performance of and Responsibility for Household Tasks: Mean Scores Reported by Well Group Couples

SOURCE: From "The Impact of Alzheimer's Disease on the Marital Relationship" by L. K. Wright, 1991, *The Gerontologist, 31*(2), p. 227. Copyright © The Gerontological Society of America. Reprinted with permission.

Adjustment Rating Scale. Handling family finances, household tasks, and other consensus issues such as making major decisions or dealing with in-laws are included in this subscale. Six response options are provided, ranging from *always agree* (6) to *always disagree* (1). The maximum consensus score on this scale is 78; the lowest is 13.

TABLE 2.1 Mean Consensus Scores by Group and Couple Comparison

	Group comparison (means)				
	Alzheimer's group			Well group	
	$n = 30$			$n = 17$	
	66			68	

		Couple comparison (means)			
Female caregiver	Male AD	Male caregiver	Female AD	Female	Male
$n = 24$	$n = 24$	$n = 6$	$n = 6$	$n = 17$	$n = 17$
67	72	64	75*	68	69

NOTE: Possible range of scores: 78 = highest consensus, 13 = lowest consensus.
*$p < .05$.

Interestingly, all spouses indicated high agreement, and no difference in level of agreement between AD and well group couples was found. As shown in Table 2.1, the means were 66 for the AD group and 68 for the well group (out of a maximum of 78).

Only when subdividing AD group couples into male afflicted/ female caregivers versus female afflicted/male caregivers did a difference emerge. Male caregivers, compared to their afflicted wives, reported significantly lower agreement (64 versus 75). Two anecdotal accounts may explain why. One caregiver husband whose afflicted wife had previously managed all finances was faced with simplifying her record keeping. For years she had recorded every item, even toothpaste, bread, milk, shoes, and large household goods, by date, where purchased, and amount paid plus tax. She wanted him to continue to "keep the books as he ought to," but he quietly had discarded many of the logs.

Another male caregiver was faced with a much more serious situation. His wife had also previously managed all family finances. Initially he had not noticed her failing memory, which resulted in unpaid insurance bills. But a young relative who had lived temporarily with the couple had noticed the woman's mental decline. Apparently he cleaned out the couple's savings account and skipped town. In essence, this couple was left without health, life, and car insurance and without something "to fall back on." It is not surprising that this male caregiver did not agree with his wife on money management. Yet he did not express anger or hostility toward her, but rather showed a quiet acceptance and a very protective demeanor toward her.

Problems Over Money Management and Coping

As the previous accounts indicate, one of the most important tasks in every marriage is the management of family finances. Monthly income had been assessed at the beginning of interview, and spouses had been asked whether they were able to meet monthly expenses for food, heating, water, clothing, and so on, and whether they could handle any unexpected major purchases such as a new refrigerator and long-term medical care. But to assess the couples' interactions and problems over money matters, two additional questions were posed: "How do you feel about your present financial arrangements?" and "Are there any problems?" Spouses were interviewed separately for these questions.

The answers given were diverse, but some important issues and common problems could be discerned. First, whether or not a change had occurred in role relationships over money management was included spontaneously in the answers. This inclusion revealed that caregivers were more likely to experience problems when the afflicted spouse had previously managed all family finances than when joint money management had been the previous pattern. But even when a total role change had occurred, a substantial number of caregivers reported no problems concerning money management; they enjoyed the control over resources that previously had been denied to them.

Those caregivers who did voice problems over money management (31%) either felt incompetent about the details of money matters or felt competent but were emotionally upset or felt emotionally drained over money matters. Some caregiver spouses (21%) were concerned over the adequacy of their financial resources, but a substantial number of caregivers (48%) experienced no problems.

TABLE 2.2 Examples of Money-Related Problems Reported by AD Couples

Caregiver spouses

Role change

"In lots of ways it does cause problems for me; it's lots of responsibility; he used to carry it all, but now all this paper . . ."

"We need to do it together; I have done it for 5 years now; it doesn't bother me."

Competency issues

"It bothers me. I am not experienced in stocks and all those things."

"It has caused considerable problems; I had to learn from scratch."

Emotional issues

"I'm adequate at it, but I get despondent. We used to do it together."

"Mentally I get tired having to make all the decisions; but he used to be in full control. My life is comfortable now."

Financial adequacy issues

"I had to file for bankruptcy since he lost his income."

"If he has to go into a nursing home, I will lose my house. What will happen to me?"

"I feel I can't spend money on clothing or on a vacation; what little we have saved, we may need later when he is sicker."

No problems

"I think I'm doing real well. Grew into it."

"I feel competent. I have always known how to handle money."

"Never liked it but always done it."

"I didn't do it before. It was a gradual process. I do it all now. I kind of enjoy learning it. He used to be real secretive, and I had to just take whatever he wanted (me to have)."

Caregiver spouses' innovative strategies to involve the afflicted spouse

"I prepare the checks but let him put his signature on the checks."

"I still ask his opinion when I want to buy something."

"I let him have his own pension so he can pay for the groceries."

"I will ask him to write specific checks, and he will do it."

"When we go out to eat, I give him money so he can pay for it."

continued

A sampling of typical answers from caregiver and afflicted spouses is presented in Table 2.2. The answers are grouped according to the issues or problems identified.

TABLE 2.2 Continued

Afflicted spouses

Role change
   "I want to know what he is doing." (Had previously managed the money)
Competency issues
   None voiced.
Emotional issues
   "It's frustrating at times. He doesn't keep the books as he ought to."
Veiled problem statements
   "Okay with me as long as she does what I want (laughs). As long as
   outsiders don't get into it."
   "She does it pretty well (pause); she spends money on the grandchildren."
   "Have to accept it (pause). He sold some silver coins."
Financial adequacy issues
   None voiced.
No problems
   "Doesn't trouble me if it doesn't trouble her."
   "No, I have no problem with her handling it all."
   "I get the money and she spends it, That's what I married her for."
   "Doesn't bother me."
   "Okay with me. She always handled the money."
   "She doesn't steal it from me. It takes a lot off my mind."
   "I want her to handle it. She is more capable than I."
   "She is conservative. She is good with money."
   "I don't want to bother; she is the best I've ever known."
   "It's great that he does it. He has always done it."

It is also interesting to note that several caregiver wives (17%) made special efforts to keep their husbands involved in money matters through such strategies as preparing the checks but letting him sign them (see Table 2.2). In this way they tried to preserve the illusion of involvement.

When focusing on the afflicted spouses' answers (Table 2.2), the dominant theme was denial of problems over money; only the female spouse who had kept detailed purchase records openly voiced frustration. In addition, a few afflicted spouses made veiled comments about being displeased; these spouses seemed to acquiesce rather than confront the issue. All other afflicted spouses stated, often in rather constricted and cryptic language, that they were not troubled over money management even in cases where the caregiver was experiencing problems. However, several of the afflicted spouses quite accurately commented on their spouses' competence in money matters.

The questions "How do you feel about your present financial arrangements?" and "Are there any problems?" were also put to the well group spouses. Typical answers are listed in Table 2.3.

Interestingly quite a large number of well group couples (59%) voiced problems over money management, but for these couples most problems occurred when money was managed together, not because they had to do it alone. Female spouses were more likely to voice concern over competency issues, while emotional aspects—often an intense dislike for the time it takes to handle money—were shared about equally between husbands and wives. Yet only 6% of couples in this comparison group mentioned problems over financial resources (both spouses mentioned it), in contrast to 21% of caregiver spouses. The mean monthly income for well couples was $2,073, and $1,862 for AD couples; statistically the difference is not significant, supporting the finding by other researchers that financial resources of AD couples tend to be similar to those in the general population (Dura, Haywood-Niler, & Kiecolt-Glaser, 1990; George & Gwyther, 1986). However, in this study couples were questioned not only about combined monthly income but also about whether they were able to meet regular household expenses, a major purchase, and long-term care. This detailed questioning may have brought out the difference over perceived financial adequacy.

It is important to note, however, that a considerable proportion of both groups reported no problems: 48% of caregiver spouses and 35% of well group spouses. A summary of problems encountered by both groups is presented in Table 2.4.

TABLE 2.3 Examples of Money-Related Problems Reported by Well Couples

---

Female spouses

Role changes

"I'm trying to show him."

"I tell him I should know, but (I) keep putting it off."

Competence issues

"I would be absolutely lost if I had to handle the money."

"I'm beginning to look at it, but the taxes are overwhelming."

Emotional issues

"I feel competent handling the money; he is the one who jumped into things."

"We try to come to some agreement with discussions."

Financial adequacy issues

"We do it together. If I had to, I could handle it. We know what comes in."

"No, we wouldn't have enough money for really big household expenses."

No problems

"No problems because there are no secrets between us."

"I've always done it: I don't mind doing the books. I get things ready, and he signs the checks. This doesn't mean I cannot sign, I do so quite often, but letting him sign is a way of keeping him involved so that he knows what's going on."

Male spouses

Role changes

"Present arrangement is working fine; she is now learning."

Competency issues

None voiced.

Emotional issues

"It's okay with me that she handles it. The only thing we haven't settled on is the will. I have left all to her. She won't tell me if she has done the same for me."

"I like it to be different than it is now, that she handles hers and I mine—because of the children (second marriage for both). It's impossible to teach her, she doesn't know math."

Financial adequacy issues

"There is no disagreement; we tell each other what we can spend . . . . No, we wouldn't have enough for big household emergencies."

No problems

"No problems there. I have always done it."

TABLE 2.4 Summary of Money-Related Problems by Caregiver and Well Group Spouses

Problem	Caregivers[a]		Well spouses	
	n	%	n	%
No problems	14	48	12	35
Competence and/or emotional problems	9	31	20	59
Resources or adequacy problems	6	21	2	6
Total	29	100	34	100

SOURCE: From "The Impact of Alzheimer's Disease on the Marital Relationship" by L. K. Wright, 1991, *The Gerontologist, 31*(2), p. 231. Copyright © The Gerontological Society of America. Reprinted with permission.
NOTE: a. In addition to the caregiver spouses' stated problems, one female AD spouse voiced frustration, and five other afflicted spouses (four males, one female) made veiled problem statements; see Table 2.2.

HUMAN DEVELOPMENT AND HOUSEHOLD TASKS OF MARRIAGE

What do these findings tell us about human development? For well spouses, responsibilities for instrumental or household tasks are played out between sociocultural and psychological life dimensions—that is, between the "oughts" of gender roles and individual psychological expectations. If conflicts arise, outcomes for well couples can be exploitation or acculturation (Riegel, 1976). For Alzheimer's couples, conflicts arise because of biological limitations in the afflicted spouse and sociocultural demands placed on the caregiver spouse or the caregiver's own expectations. For these couples the outcomes can be adaptation or distortion (Riegel, 1976).

As previously discussed and shown in Figure 2.2, well group spouses share financial management. This is a striking finding, considering that the mean age of these couples was 70 years and that most were retired. Hertz (1986) reported that among younger, well-paid dual-career couples, separate accounts and joint financial responsibilities are an emerging pattern, but for working-class and professional middle-class families, the husband still manages the money and makes major financial decisions.

Nevertheless over a 40-year period a change in marital attitudes over family finances seems to have occurred. In 1940 Holahan (1984) examined attitudes concerning money held by a group of married couples who were then in their 30s. In 1980 the same couples, who were now in their 70s, were questioned again. Their attitudes concerning money had changed. Holahan (1984) then contrasted those new attitudes with answers from a contemporary, young group of couples. This tactic showed that by 1980 the older couples held attitudes similar to those of the contemporary group. For example, both groups indicated that the wife should have greater financial involvement in money management. Culturally the older couples in Holahan's study had been assimilated into contemporary marriage roles.

But in addition to cultural attitude changes, the sharing of money responsibilities among well couples in this sample may also be explained from a life span developmental perspective. Those spouses, male and female alike, who at present were managing most or all of the money were making efforts to involve and teach their respective mates, and a number of couples had evolved into a pattern of alternating the task of paying monthly bills. Both partners seemed to recognize the need for such involvement. Their strategies reflect a sense of preparing the other spouse for widowhood. Even though a devastating illness was not present, the biological clock was taken into consideration. The couples' answers reflect life span developmental thinking and adaptation rather than changes in cultural attitudes.

Management of money in the presence of Alzheimer's disease, however, is quite different. In fact, none of the Alzheimer's afflicted spouses any longer managed finances totally by themselves or carried total responsibility for financial matters. In most instances not even a sharing of responsibilities developed. Previous research findings concerning quantitative increase in caregiver responsibilities are clearly supported (Kapust, 1982; Miller, 1987; Stone et al., 1987; Zarit, Todd, & Zarit, 1986). The five instances in which female caregiver spouses had found innovative ways of involving an ill husband were different from the involvement reported by spouses in the well group. In the AD group the caregiver spouse took on a worried, supervisory tone; it was not an involvement in which both could grow in knowledge, but rather a one-sided, protective maneuver motivated perhaps by not fully accepting or giving in to the spouse's deterioration. Miller (1987) reported similar strategies used by caregiver wives in an effort to maintain the husbands' self-esteem. Miller (1987) suggested that such caregiver wives draw on their previous repertoire of support-oriented behaviors; they seek a balance between previous marital role relationships and the new situation of being in control. But as shown in this study, a large percentage of caregivers adapt well to being in control; their comments reflect a gain in confidence and competence.

The denial of problems over money by most afflicted spouses is particularly interesting when viewed from a developmental perspective. Afflicted spouses had a distorted "definition of the situation," and even when the caregiver spouses had problems, they were unable to recognize them or to "take the attitude of the other." The perceived absence of problems was not developmental adaptation, but rather distortion of their environment (Riegel, 1976).

According to the theoretical formulations of this book, problems or life difficulties (asynchronies) are major determinants of development. Well group couples actually experience more problems over money management than the caregivers, and most of the well couples' problems occur when they interact. Hence relatively healthy couples have more opportunity for development. But cognitively impaired Alzheimer's persons no longer perceive problems or asynchronies, and thus their development ceases. Nevertheless they are part of a dyadic relationship, and their presence facilitates transformations in the caregiver spouse. The transformations in this case are the significantly increased responsibilities and the caregivers' quite remarkable adaptation, indicating developmental growth in coping with often new and complex issues.

ASSESSMENT STRATEGIES AND INTERVENTION GUIDELINES

Based on findings from this study, as well as findings and recommendations from other researchers, several assessment strategies and intervention guidelines are offered.

Assessment Strategies

Health professionals and also caregivers themselves can use several strategies for assessing the management of household tasks when one spouse has Alzheimer's disease. Important questions are (a) Who is in charge of money matters? (b) Has legal counsel for long-term money arrangements been obtained? (c) Who does what task? and (d) How do you feel about handling those tasks, and what problems have you encountered? For the "Who does what task?" question, the scale shown in Figure 2.1 may be used. It assesses who does which specific household chore and who is responsible for making sure that each gets done. The responses range was *I never do it* = 1; *I rarely do it* = 2; *I do it about half of the time* = 3; *I do it most of the time* = 4; *I do it all the time* = 5. Cue cards with the options in large, bold print are helpful, particularly if the information also is sought from afflicted spouses. Finally each spouse may be asked to identify feelings and specific problems concerning specific tasks.

Intervention Guidelines

Just by asking "Who is in charge of money matters?" intervention has begun because it draws attention to one of the most crucial issues faced by caregiver spouses. Even if there is only the suspicion of memory loss, the spouse without memory problems, if not already in charge, must take over the handling of money matters immediately. Some of the innovative strategies developed by caregivers can be used to maintain the afflicted spouses' self-esteem (see Table 2.2).

The issue of who is in charge of money needs to be raised every time clinicians and researchers address audiences, particularly with older couples present. We can learn from the experiences of AD couples and also from the evolving role relationships reported by well couples in this study. When both spouses are involved in money management, some of the most devastating losses experienced by AD couples can be prevented. Every couple needs to be encouraged to share in money management even if both spouses are perfectly healthy. It seems such simple advice, but it takes deliberate commitment and effort to do so. Encouragement to make specific plans for teaching each other must be given. An excellent suggestion is to take turns paying the monthly bills, a strategy developed by the well couples in this study. Bank accounts that list both spouses' names with an *or* notation are recommended over the *and* notation; when needed, *or* allows one spouse (the well spouse, it is hoped) access to and control over assets.

The next question, "Has legal counsel for long-range money arrangements been obtained?" is equally crucial when one spouse has memory problems. Caregivers may be reluctant to seek legal advice in the early stages of the spouses' illness, thinking that such a step means they are declaring the spouses "incompetent." This is not the case. Rather, early legal advice can prevent many money-related difficulties as the disease progresses. An attorney can, for example, advise that the afflicted spouse, while still capable, grant durable power of attorney to the caregiver spouse (instead of simple power of attorney). This means that even when the afflicted spouse later becomes incompetent, the arrangements made under durable power of attorney are still valid (Overman & Stoudemire, 1988). Durable power of attorney also can prevent the lengthy and costly procedures of guardianship that may have to be implemented if plans have not been made while the afflicted spouse still has the capacity to understand and sign documents (Overman & Stoudemire, 1988). In addition, the caregiver can discuss with an attorney long-range plans for eventual institutionalization. This may be a painful topic to address for caregivers, but health professionals need to encourage caregivers to seek such advice. Misconceptions may need to be cleared up: It is quite common that caregivers expect Medicare to pay for eventual nursing home care or believe that they, the caregivers, will invariably lose their homes; neither is true. A more detailed discussion concerning Medicare and Medicaid can be found in Chapter 6.

Considering the importance of financial arrangements in the early stages of the illness, it is necessary that caregivers ask for a tentative diagnosis when talking to the ill spouse's physician and then seek legal counsel. The local Alzheimer's Association (the local chapter of the Alzheimer's Disease and Related Disorders Association, or ADRDA) has names of attorneys who specialize in such legal matters. Almost every state has a local chapter; if you cannot find the phone number, the National Headquarters of the Alzheimer's Association may be contacted at 919 North Michigan Avenue, Suite 1000, Chicago, IL 60611-1676, (800) 272-3900.

The "Who does what task?" scale provides a quick assessment of current role relationships between husband and wife, as well as an assessment of afflicted spouses' functional abilities. In addition, health care professionals and caregiver spouses may use the scale to assess which tasks an afflicted spouse can perform safely. For example, cleaning up the table after a meal, cleaning a floor, or dusting furniture are relatively safe tasks, but cooking may be unsafe. Yet it is important that a couple retain normal role relationships as much as possible and maximize the afflicted spouse's abilities. This strategy requires the caregiver to use some very specific communication skills (Beck & Heacock, 1988; Farran & Keane-Hagerty, 1989; Hall, 1988; Harvis, 1990). For example, the caregiver spouse can look at the afflicted spouse directly, point to the table (or chair, or corner of the room), and say, "I need your help. Please stack the magazines over there." Afflicted spouses in the early and even middle stages of Alzheimer's disease can follow such simple one-step requests and thus can experience success and self-worth. Caregivers must avoid "You can't do this . . . " statements; they increase the afflicted spouse's frustration and sense of failure.

Going grocery shopping together is relatively safe, but the caregiver needs to reevaluate this activity from time to time to determine whether it is too stimulating for the afflicted spouse and whether it leads to increased agitation (Hall, 1988). Choosing times when stores are relatively empty is a good strategy. Once in the store, simple instructions for what to pick off the shelf should be used. For example, the caregiver spouse can point to a specific cereal box and say, "That's the one. Put it in the cart." This is a two-step command; if the afflicted spouse has trouble completing the entire task, one-step commands may be given (Heacock, Walton, Beck, & Mercer, 1991). For example, the caregiver can point and say, "That's the one." When the box is in the afflicted spouse's hand, the caregiver can make the next request, "Now put it in the cart." These strategies will keep the afflicted spouse involved in tasks; at the same time, these strategies facilitate day-to-day interactions between couples, and interactions are to be encouraged. As Heacock et al. (1991) observed, when interactions with the environment cease, afflicted persons begin to interact with themselves through rocking, moaning, and mumbling.

Questioning both spouses about feelings concerning household tasks provides good information about current problem areas and also about past role relationships. Questioning also brings to light whether a caregiver spouse feels fatigued and helpless in specific areas. Interventions can, for example, be focused on arranging for help with managing money. Usually the caregiver can identify a trusted family member who can be approached to provide assistance. Interventions also may be focused on providing the caregiver with relief from household tasks, either because the tasks are physically too demanding or because the caregiver just needs to get away. Health care professionals need to discuss options available to caregivers and to individualize the needed help (Baldwin, 1988, 1990). The local Alzheimer's Association is an excellent resource for arranging suitable and affordable respite care. Probably the most important message to convey to caregivers is that much has been learned from others who faced similar situations and that, today, help is available (Baldwin, 1990).

Tension Within the Marital Relationship

INTRODUCTION

Every couple will experience some tension as part of their marriage relationship; however, high tension in the form of frequent quarrels, constantly getting on each other's nerves, and frequent thoughts of leaving are a threat to the marriage relationship and could signal its impending termination. The tension dimension captures the partners' negative interactions with each other and the emergent quality of development. The extent to which spouses are able to "take the attitude of the other" and how they "define the situation" becomes important in reducing tension.

EXPLORING TENSION

Tension between spouses was explored with three major questions: (a) What causes tension? (b) What level of tension do both groups of couples report, and are husbands and wives similar or different in their assessment of tension? and (c) How do couples cope with tension?

What Causes Tension?

Each spouse was asked to describe in his or her own words situations that cause tension. The topic was introduced by saying, "All couples will quarrel sometime. Can you tell me what you and your spouse quarrel about?" Another question was "What does your spouse do that gets on your nerves?" Spouses were interviewed separately for these questions.

Typical answers given by AD and well group spouses are shown in Tables 3.1 and 3.2. The responses reveal that caregivers focused exclusively on the illness context—that is, how the disease affected the relationship. The afflicted spouses' repetitive questioning and restless walking, their verbal abuse, and the need to give repeated instructions were named as sources of tension and aggravation by caregivers. However, 40% of all afflicted spouses defined the situation as nonproblematic; they claimed no real problems between them and their spouse.

Well group couples did not have one focal point of tension, but rather named a number of situations ranging from quarrels over church attendance, travel, relatives, and their grown children to cooking and kitchen chores. Sometimes the other spouse's physical limitation or emotional state also was mentioned as a source of tension—for example, walking very slowly or the partner's depressed moods.

For both groups, however, there was evidence of "taking the attitude of the other," of interpreting the spouse's actions, remarks, and feelings. Couples seemed to sense what the other spouse thought or felt, and this influenced their subsequent actions. A good example is the comment by one caregiver spouse: "I get on his (nerves), and he gets on mine because he can't do anything right. . . . but I talk to myself a lot. Right now, he is real sweet, he tries to please me. . . . " This caregiver spouse is not only aware of her own frustration but also acknowledges his attempt to please her. Instead of getting mad at him, she talks to herself.

Although such awareness is perhaps not too surprising in caregivers, the finding that 33% of all afflicted spouses showed similar awareness is remarkable. A female afflicted spouse's

TABLE 3.1 Examples of Tension-Causing Situations Reported by AD Couples

---

Caregiver spouses

Female caregivers

"I get on his (nerves), and he gets on mine because he can't do anything right. I have to go behind him on everything. But I talk to myself a lot. Right now, he is real sweet and kind; he tries to please me and give me space."

"He loves to go out. He wants to go somewhere all the time. I get some rest when I take him to the day-care center. But some days he doesn't want to go."

"I have to give him step-by-step instructions, very patiently; I have to explain things for 10 minutes; it exhausts my patience."

"Last Saturday, I told my daughter, 'Get me out of here.' He really got to me. He walks all day. I had the flu, I couldn't escape."

"He will say to me, 'You have been through hell today.' I noticed that he will go for a walk when we quarrel over what he can no longer do."

"Sometimes he gets very frustrated, and then he is cursing; (he) almost hit me, so the doctor put him on Mellaril. He abuses me verbally."

Male caregiver

"It gets on my nerves when she can't remember."

Afflicted spouses

Male afflicted

"Naturally (we get on each other's nerves), but not very often. I go for a walk then, stretch my legs; there is no objection to it, and she gets some benefit from it."

"I get on her nerves, but we settle it. Well, I go out in the yard, piddle around, it takes up time."

"All these people, they play (referring to wife's bridge group). I just let them do it and go into the yard."

Female afflicted

"Sometimes I get mad, but I keep quiet so he doesn't get mad."

---

comment "Sometimes I get mad, but I keep quiet so he doesn't get mad" is an example.

High awareness by well spouses is epitomized by the statement "I don't know, we just sense each other." This "sensing" influenced subsequent actions, as indicated by these words: "If the other doesn't care (to do something), usually one gives in" (see Table 3.2).

TABLE 3.2 Examples of Tension-Causing Situations Reported by
Well Couples

Female spouses

"I'm not as much of a TV bug as he is, so I try to find something else to do
and leave the room. We may not even have had a word about it."

"I learned if you say things, you can't take it back. I storm and he pouts.
Lots of times I feel that he is hurt, and I ask him to forgive me because I
say things, and they injure him."

"The biggest problem is all those trips he wants to take. I fuss but give in;
he always wins out."

"I fuss, and he is real quiet. If I had a complaint about him, it's that he
internalizes a lot and I talk too much."

"I don't know, we just sense each other; if the other doesn't care (to do
something), usually one gives in."

"If we can't do something (because of his walking difficulties) and I get
disappointed, I try to keep it from showing. If he says, 'Honey, I hold you
back,' I say, 'Oh, no, I'm very happy.' "

Male spouses

"We don't have real big arguments that often. After you have lived with a
person for more than 30 years, you know what creates problems, you just
try to avoid those."

"I don't want to win points. She is more the one who wants to make a
point. It's just a matter of reexamining oneself, try to understand the other
person's outlook versus mine."

"We probably all have some selfishness. I may insist on something, and
she gives in more than I do, and I appreciate that. But maybe she has me
trained to think she is giving in."

"Our main disagreement is that she likes to travel and I don't care about
it. I don't like shopping either, but she doesn't insist."

"Well, she's more religious than I; I don't like to go to church twice on
Sundays. She pushes me into that, but I go along with some coaxing."

"When something is overcooked, I comment on it and that's the end of it."

What Is the Level of Tension?

To assess perceived level of tension between spouses, the
tension subscale of Spanier and Thompson's (1982) Dyadic
Adjustment Rating Scale was used. Frequency of quarreling,
getting on each other's nerves, leaving after a fight, regretting
having married, and considering or discussing divorce, separa-

TABLE 3.3 Mean Tension Scores by Group and Couple Comparison

Group comparison (means)					
Alzheimer's group				*Well group*	
n = 30				*n* = 17	
25				27	
		Couple comparison (means)			
Female caregiver	*Male AD*	*Male caregiver*	*Female AD*	*Female*	*Male*
n = 24	*n* = 24	*n* = 6	*n* = 6	*n* = 17	*n* = 17
25	28*	25	25	26	27

NOTE: Possible range of scores: 30 = lowest tension, 5 = highest tension.
*$p < .01$.

tion, or termination of the relationship are questioned with this scale. Response options range from *never* (6) to *all the time* (1). It should be noted that in this case a high score indicates low tension. The maximum score, representing lowest tension, is 30; a score of 5 indicates very high tension.

Spouses generally reported low tension on this scale. As shown in Table 3.3, there was no significant difference in level of tension between the AD and well group, no difference between husbands and wives from the well group, and no difference between couples comprised of male caregivers and female afflicted spouses. Male afflicted spouses, however, assessed their tension level as significantly lower than the female caregivers (a mean of 28 versus 25, with the higher score indicating lower tension).

The lower tension level by male afflicted spouses is quite consistent with their denial of problems when they had been asked to describe tension. However, even the female caregivers' tension levels were quite low and very similar to those of other spouse dyads. Yet tension had most definitely been reported by caregiver spouses and also by well group spouses when they were asked to describe specific situations (see Table 3.1 and Table 3.2). So why did they rate their tension as low on the scale? This question will be explored next.

How Do Couples Cope With Tension?

Spouses were asked to describe how they dealt with trouble-some situations described by them. Typical answers are presented in Table 3.4 for the AD group and Table 3.5 for the well group. Responses from caregiver spouses reflect intense emotional control and release of anguish by displacing it onto a different target: screaming into a pillow, grabbing the bathroom sink, or rifle shooting, for example. Unsuccessful control of tension tended to create feelings of guilt. These spouses knew they "should not" get angry, should not according to society's standards and widely publicized caregiver manuals that have defined ill persons as not responsible for their actions (Baldwin, 1990). Mead's (1977) *generalized other,* the attitude of the whole community, is exemplified here: It directs the thoughts and actions of the caregiver spouses.

Limit setting, diversion, and removing themselves from the situation were additional coping strategies used by caregivers. Only a few reported that they still openly expressed their feelings to their spouses. Most caregiver spouses compensated this loss of open communication with other coping strategies. Yet keeping control of the situation seemed to be the purpose of all of these actions. The initial contradiction between the caregivers' descriptions of feeling high tension but rating expression of tension as low on the scale now becomes clear: Tension was rated as low because caregivers made intense efforts to keep it low. The full meaning of their situation comes into focus when combining qualitative and quantitative assessments of tension.

A summary of coping strategies used to reduce tension is shown in Figure 3.1. Frequency counts indicate that intense emotional control was used by 33% of caregiver spouses, diversion by 23%, limit setting by 10%, keeping quiet by 7%, and removing oneself from the situation also by 7%. Only 13% still openly expressed their feelings to their spouses.

For afflicted spouses, predominant strategies for reducing tension were defining the situation as nonproblematic (40%) and removing themselves from conflict (33%). Only four (13%) afflicted spouses stated that they still "argued it out." Four others indicated

TABLE 3.4 Examples of Coping With Tension Reported by AD Couples

---

Caregiver spouses

Female caregivers

> "When we quarrel, I just go to the bathroom. I have privacy there, and I grab the sink and say, 'God, help me.' And I cry."

> "You have to treat him like a child and set strict limits. It works, it quiets him down. You have to be a strong person or it would have killed me or both."

> "Sometimes I go to the bedroom and scream into a pillow and then come out and carry on. And I laugh a lot about things that aren't laughable. I seldom cry, though this morning I did."

> "I put up with it (repeated questions) as long as possible without screaming, but then I blow my stack and start screaming. I know I shouldn't, you're always sorry afterwards. I stop and remind myself that it's not his fault, but anger is a big part of it. I have to stop and get control."

> "I try not to get mad, but if people hurt you so bad, you want to lash out."

> "I pray for strength and patience all the time. Sometimes I scream at him, I know I shouldn't, and I feel guilty, and then I go for a walk."

> "When he gets on my nerves, I walk away, read, go upstairs, or shopping, get out of the house."

Male caregivers

> "When she gets on my nerves, I just accept it, the source, and don't let it bother me. That's the only way it can be handled. If there is an argument, I change the conversation. I ignore it."

> "I try to get some shooting in at the club. It gets the aggression out. You feel tired afterwards."

Afflicted spouses

Male afflicted

> "It happens very rarely (getting on each other's nerves); if it happens, I go outside."

> "Years ago, I wouldn't have handled it good. Now I smooth it over. I believe I can hold my temper now so it won't hurt anyone. I kind of quieted down."

> "We argue it out."

> "I laugh and walk off."

> "I overlook it and keep going."

> "We have no problems."

> "We don't quarrel."

> "Just a little cat scratch."

Female afflicted

> "When he gets on my nerves, I try to keep my mouth shut; it works. It doesn't last long."

TABLE 3.5 Examples of Coping With Tension Reported by Well Couples

Female spouses

"I say what I want to say, and he says what he wants. That's the end of it; there is no pouting."

"There are two of us. I got a right to express myself and I do. No one wins. Ten to 15 minutes go by, and then it's past history."

"I tend to get into my shell; he is the opposite, keeps at it until it is out in the open. It clears the air."

"He used to clam up, but now we talk about it. He is so sweet and easygoing."

"I spew off for a while and then shut up; there are no big fights, though."

Male spouses

"If I disagree with the wife, we reason it out."

"We are open, we're never falling asleep still angry with each other. Mutual respect has been good for 45 years."

"Usually we say what we want to say, let the chips fall and go about our other activities. Neither of us is very argumentative; we don't harass each other because of disagreements. She will tell me I'm hard headed, and that's the end of the discussion. We handle it pretty well. Things rarely carry over into the next day."

"The main thing is to go back and admit that you were wrong or took the wrong attitude in an effort to reconcile."

"I mainly shut up and give it the silent treatment. Fifteen years ago, I may have left the house, but not now. We get along real well, the longer the better."

---

that they held their temper and kept quiet. None of the afflicted spouses, however, used the intense emotional control reported by their caregiver spouses. The actions by afflicted spouses seemed to serve a dual purpose: to avoid discordance and to prevent disorder. They avoided discordance through denial of problems and acquiescence. Thus they indirectly were able to keep some control over the situation and prevent total disorder.

A different pattern emerged for the well group couples. The predominant strategy for dealing with tension was expressing oneself to or confronting the spouse. It was used by 53% of well group couples, in contrast to only 13% of AD group couples. Keeping quiet and removing oneself from the situation were used by 47% of well group couples, but intense emotional control, limit setting,

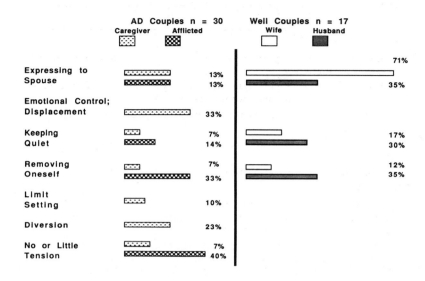

Figure 3.1. Coping With Tension: Alzheimer's and Well Couples Percentage of Time Strategies Were Used*

and diversion as used by caregivers did not occur. Wives from the well group used open expression twice as often as their spouses (71% wives versus 35% husbands). Husbands were more likely to keep quiet and to remove themselves from the situation (65% husbands versus 29% wives). But all spouses from the well group mentioned that they could somehow reach agreement. They expressed confidence that even if the other one was "spouting off," harmony, or concordance, could be restored. Most likely this is the reason why, despite the well group couples' descriptions of a number of tension-producing situations, their scores on the quantitated scale showed such low tension.

HUMAN DEVELOPMENT
AND MARITAL TENSION

Findings about tension have implications for human development. For couples in the AD group, tension results from asynchronies between the afflicted spouse's biological and both partners' psychological life dimensions. For well group couples, tension is played out between the husband's and wife's intersecting psychological dimensions (Riegel, 1976; Wright, 1989; see Table 1.1). In this study the experience of tension is indeed different for the two groups. Coping strategies described by caregiver spouses reflect a need to keep control, and efforts are directed at preventing disorder; although handled differently, this need is echoed by their afflicted mates. Well group couples, however, no matter how tension is handled, always included a statement of being very confident that they can work things out. In other words, they can reach concordance (Riegel, 1976). The possibility exists, of course, that only couples with harmonious relationships consented to be interviewed. Yet in general, research supports that the later years of the life cycle bring increased marital happiness (Gilford, 1984; Spanier, Lewis, & Cole, 1975; Weishaus & Field, 1988).

In this study wives from the well group evidenced high emotional expressiveness. Similar findings have been reported by Neugarten and Gutmann (1958) and Feldman, Biringen, and Nash (1981), who documented increased dominance and aggressiveness in older married women, while older men tended to become more acquiescent.

A particularly interesting finding in this study is that proportionally as many well group husbands as Alzheimer's afflicted husbands reported that they remove themselves from tense situations (35% versus 33%, respectively). Only one female afflicted spouse reported doing this. Perhaps, then, this strategy of minimizing tension can, in part, be explained as a gender and developmental phenomenon. Some support for this interpretation is found in the study by Quayhagen and Quayhagen (1988), who reported that a coping strategy called *minimizing the threat* was positively related to existential growth for caregivers. However, husbands and wives in Quayhagen & Quayhagen's study were not different in their use of minimizing the threat.

Even more important is the finding that 40% of afflicted spouses claimed absence of problems. This finding is congruent with their assessment of consensus over household tasks described in Chapter 2. Denial of problems can be interpreted as the afflicted spouses' attempts to simplify the environment and thus to maintain some control over surroundings. The continuing need by afflicted persons to control their environment also has been described by Beck and Heacock (1988). Denial of problems thus may be adaptive; yet at the same time, it points to the deteriorating cognitive functioning and the tentative explanation that when the ability to perceive asynchronies is lost, development ceases.

In summary, control is the dominant coping strategy used for reducing tension in the Alzheimer's group, and the goal is to prevent total disorder. Confrontation is the dominant strategy for reducing tension among well group couples, and the goal is to reach concordance. These outcomes support Riegel's (1976) propositions.

ASSESSMENT STRATEGIES AND INTERVENTION GUIDELINES

Findings from this study and reports from other researchers concerning tension provide the basis for assessment strategies and intervention guidelines offered to health professionals and caregivers. Because prolonged efforts to keep high tension under control can adversely affect health, tension assessment needs to include questions about the caregivers' emotional and physical health.

Assessment Strategies

Four important issues need to be assessed: (a) Is tension openly expressed between spouses? (b) What specifically produces tension? (c) How does the caregiver handle tension? and (d) When does the caregiver need to be referred for individual counseling? The following questions will elicit the needed information: "Do you and your spouse quarrel?" "What do you quarrel about?"

"What does your spouse do that gets on your nerves?" "How do you handle such situations?" "How distressed and how depressed do you feel?" "Has your health been affected by this tension?" "Have you given up on him or her?" The last question may be supplemented with an assessment of commitment to the spouse as a valued person (refer to Chapter 6).

Intervention Guidelines

All questions must be posed in an unhurried manner and convey to caregivers that they have the health professional's undivided attention. The question "Do you and your spouse quarrel?" is important because a negative reply may indicate that the afflicted spouse is quite passive and easy to be with; on the other hand, it may indicate that the caregiver uses intense self-control to avoid quarrels. If the answer is affirmative, then the next question, "What do you quarrel about?" will elicit descriptions of specific situations; if quarrels are denied, then the question "What does your spouse do that gets on your nerves?" will elicit the caregiver's subjective experience of tension. Caregivers are likely to focus on their most intense emotional experiences, and as they describe specific incidents, they may also be asked "How do you handle such situations?" At this point in the questioning, the health professional should focus on interventions for managing the afflicted spouse's behavior but mentally make a note to address interventions for the caregiver's distress later.

Specific behavior problems will require specific interventions, but frequently mentioned problems are restless wandering, agitation and frustration or "getting mad over nothing," along with verbal abuse, which has the potential of escalating into physical abuse.

Helping the caregiver understand the meaning of wandering is the health professional's task. The afflicted spouse's wandering may be the lifelong pattern of a very active person who used activity or walking to cope with stress (Beck & Heacock, 1988). But wandering also may be a search for safety and belonging or some other felt need; this type of wandering has been termed *agenda behavior* (Beck & Heacock, 1988). If the afflicted spouse was a very industrious person in the past, then structured physical exercise or household tasks congruent with previous responsibilities may help reduce wandering. But if wandering seems to be a search for something, then the wanderer's mood can provide some clues to his or her felt need, or "agenda." For example, an afflicted spouse's hasty attempt to leave and the comment "I have to visit mother's house" may be an attempt to recapture old satisfying situations (Beck & Heacock, 1988). It is helpful to respond to that implied need and to acknowledge it with, for example, "It's important for you to see mother's house. We need to go and visit." Then the afflicted spouse's attention can be redirected. Such strategies can prevent agitated and combative behavior. Conversely, by not responding to the implied need ("Don't be silly, mother lives 200 miles away"), agitation is likely to escalate. Caregiver spouses know their mates well, and once they understand that wandering may be agenda behavior, they will be astute in recognizing the spouse's implied need. As appropriate, visits to old neighborhoods, historic sites, and places of worship may be arranged (Snyder, Rupprecht, Pyret, Brekhus, & Moss, 1978).

Agitation and frustration are other frequently mentioned tension-producing situations. Health professionals need to assist caregivers with rating the most disturbing behaviors that require interventions and also with individualizing approaches discussed in caregiver manuals (Baldwin, 1988). However, all caregivers can be taught how to use distraction, one of the key strategies to reduce and even prevent tense encounters (Beck & Heacock, 1988; Beck, Heacock, Mercer, Walton, & Shook, 1991; Hall, 1988). To prevent verbal abuse by an agitated, frustrated afflicted spouse escalating into physical abuse, caregivers may apply the following principles: (a) Acknowledge in a calm voice that they hear or see what is bothering the spouse, (b) redirect the spouse to a different environment or change visual cues, and (c) ask a simple question to introduce a new and calming topic. For example, a caregiver could say to an agitated and frustrated spouse who has trouble getting his jacket zipped: "Yes, that zipper gets stuck a lot. Maybe it's old" (acknowledgment).

"Let's go to the kitchen (redirection). Would you like some juice?" (simple question requiring only a yes or no response; new topic). Instead of redirecting the spouse to a different room, the caregiver also could walk to the window, point outside, and say: "Let's look out of the window" (verbal communication is reinforced by nonverbal gestures, and a new visual cue is given). "It rained today. Can you see all those puddles?" (new topic; simple question). The zipper, by the way, can be adjusted later or changed to Velcro fasteners.

Next it is important to focus on the caregiver's well-being. Caregivers need to be affirmed in their efforts to keep tension between themselves and their afflicted spouses at low levels. At the same time, however, health professionals need to convey that such vigilant strategies can take their toll on the caregivers' emotional and physical health. Given, Collins, and Given (1988) suggested questioning positive reactions to caregiving, in addition to negative reactions. This questioning provides a more balanced view of the situation and also helps caregivers evaluate themselves when the next two questions are posed: "How distressed do you feel?" and "How depressed do you feel?" Caregivers who rate themselves as very distressed and score 7 or higher on a scale of 1 = *not at all depressed* to 10 = *extremely depressed* require more in-depth assessment and may need to be referred for individual counseling. In addition, the question "Has your health been affected as a result of caregiving?" is important and can lead to encouraging caregivers to seek medical attention (Given et al., 1988). When referrals to a mental health professional or to a medical practitioner are made, it is also important to arrange for appropriate supervision for the afflicted spouse so that the caregiver can keep the appointment(s). How much self-control the caregiver is exerting will have become apparent with the previous assessment strategies. The question "Have you given up on him or her?" will provide additional clues. Beck and Phillips (1983) noted that some caregivers give up on the way an afflicted person used to be as a way of coping with loss but that this giving up breaks emotional bonds and can lead to abusive behavior toward the afflicted person. Feelings of high tension also may be related to an unhappy past marital relationship. Indeed Robinson (1990a) found that the best predictor of wife caregiver's feelings of burden was past marital adjustment. It is appropriate, therefore, to discuss with caregivers that intense conflict and prolonged attempts to keep tension and emotions under control can lead to feelings of hopelessness and depression. Individual counseling or therapy should be recommended in situations where the caregiver has "given up." Individual therapy provides caregivers with a safe environment where they can be helped to face their feelings, learn to "reframe past grievances in their marriages" (Robinson, 1990a, p. 189), or deal with their premature grieving. And finally, in therapy caregivers can gain strength in coping with a very difficult life situation. Some caregivers will be unwilling to seek individual counseling. At a minimum, attending a local support group must be recommended. Support groups can provide helpful advice on managing difficult behaviors in the afflicted and also can help caregivers deal with feelings of guilt over losing control and "blowing their stack." Names of contact persons at local agencies and names and phone numbers of therapists (nurses, psychologists, social workers, physicians) are the types of information needed when making referrals. Information must always be given in writing (Gwyther & Matteson, 1983).

Health professionals have an obligation to report and monitor any suspected abuse. It does not seem to be a common occurrence among spouse caregivers, probably because few caregivers give up on the spouse; rather, as will be discussed in Chapter 6, they hang on to an image of the spouse as a valued person. Nevertheless abuse can happen. For all concerned, preventing abuse from occurring in the first place is the goal. Health professionals therefore need to encourage agency personnel and support group leaders to make available special counseling and separate support groups for spouse caregivers only. As will be shown in a later chapter, spouses feel uncomfortable discussing some of their problems in groups that are also attended by adult children and other family caregivers.

Companionship Within the Marital Relationship

INTRODUCTION

Marriage by its very nature provides companionship for two people. Being married and having a confidant have been reported consistently as factors contributing to well-being in older people (Chappell & Badger, 1989; Gove, Hughes, & Style, 1983; Longino & Lipman, 1981; Strain & Chappell, 1982). But whether marriage merely provides for the presence of another human being or whether two such people living together share thoughts and feelings and engage in joint activities makes a profound difference in the quality of their relationship. The quality of interactions will contribute to viewing the relationship as either desirable with a projected shared future or as oppressing and fostering wishes of escape. Yet even with difficult interactions, acceptance of the relationship can occur.

EXPLORING COMPANIONSHIP

Companionship was explored with three major questions: (a) How much companionship do both groups of couples report,

TABLE 4.1 Mean Companionship Scores by Group and Couple
Comparison

		Group comparison (means)			
		Alzheimer's group		Well group	
		$n = 30$		$n = 17$	
		20		27*	
		Couple comparison (means)			
Female		Male			
caregiver	Male AD	caregiver	Female AD	Female	Male
$n = 24$	$n = 24$	$n = 6$	$n = 6$	$n = 17$	$n = 17$
20	20	20	18	27	28

NOTE: Possible range of scores: 36 = high companionship, 6 = low companionship.
*$p < .001$.

and are husbands and wives similar or different in their reports
of companionship? (b) How do couples describe the quality of
spousal companionship? and (c) How do couples cope with
problems pertaining to companionship?

How Much Companionship Do Couples Report?

To assess frequency of companionship activities between couples, the cohesion subscale of Spanier and Thompson's (1982)
Dyadic Adjustment Rating Scale was used. Frequency of discussing something, exchanging ideas, laughing together, doing
something together outside the home, working on a project together, and confiding in each other are questioned with this
scale. Response options range from *more often than once a day* (6)
to *never* (1). Scores can range from 36 to 6, with 36 representing
very high companionship.

Responses from all spouses gave clear evidence of the impact
of Alzheimer's disease on marital companionship. As seen in
Table 4.1, mean frequency of shared activities was significantly
higher for the well group than for the AD group (27 versus 20,
respectively). Confiding in the other spouse also occurred significantly more often between couples from the well group.

Overall no significant differences were found between answers given by afflicted versus their caregiver spouses and male versus female spouses from the well group. In other words, husband and wife dyads gave congruent reports about how much companionship they had. Couples from the AD group, however, checked the indicator "laughing together" as occurring more frequently than any of the other items, although many caregiver spouses added "smile" instead of "laughing." Perhaps laughing (or smiling) indicated a way of coping for caregivers. In addition, only one afflicted husband reported that he and his wife "never" laughed together. When questioned about this, he said, "She don't think I'm funny," demonstrating how his evaluation of his wife's attitude influenced his own actions.

To determine whether laughing together was perhaps one aspect of togetherness that was similar for well versus AD group couples, a comparison was made for this indicator alone. The significant group difference held: Well group couples scored significantly higher than AD group couples. In addition, afflicted spouses scored lower than their caregiver spouses. Thus, although some laughing (or smiling) still occurred between couples in the presence of Alzheimer's disease, this type of positive communication was also much lower for them than for well group couples.

How Do Couples Describe the Quality of Spousal Companionship?

AD Couples

The loss of companionship for caregiver spouses becomes clear when one listens to their poignant descriptions and then contrasts them with the afflicted spouses' perceptions. This is what one caregiver had to say about companionship:

> We go to the movies a lot. At least he is quiet there. He does a lot of clinging, and I hold his hand a lot. I learned about "hugging therapy" the other day, and he likes it. But my life has drastically changed. I feel inadequate and guilty; everything needs some

work—the house, the yard. I do a lot of things now I didn't used to, but I don't feel the confidence. I escape with bridge from reality. I'm not suicidal, but I can see why someone would take a gun and shoot both; though he enjoys life, he doesn't hate it.

When her afflicted spouse was questioned about "doing things together," he zeroed in on his wife's bridge group and answered in an angry and resentful tone of voice:

> All these people . . . (pause) . . . they play. . . . I usually try to find out who is there and what they are doing around the house. These ladies come in (disgust in his voice) . . . I go in the garden then.

This answer parallels another afflicted spouse's resentment of his wife's bridge group:

> I rather she be here . . . (pause) . . . her bridge (shaking his head), she gets enough entertainment. Sometimes I wish she would get out of it.

Another caregiver tells this story:

> I cannot confide in him anymore. It upsets him, and he couldn't understand. We talk about simple things—what to wear, what day it is, what time it is. I have been exhausted by his repeated questions. I have to adjust to his schedule now. I wanted to work at a store for one day a week when he would play golf. But then he always decides not to play.

And this is what her husband had to say:

> A couple of guys got mad with me on the golf course because I called the wrong score. They probably thought I wanted to cheat. My wife said I should tell them, so I told them (about the memory problems), and I don't have problems anymore. Maybe I'm getting better or because they know. They will say, "No, you didn't have 5 or 6," and I feel better.

Not only loss of mutually satisfying companionship becomes apparent in the caregivers' accounts but also high dependency and demands for full attention by afflicted spouses. One caregiver described it as "clinging" behavior. The afflicted spouses' comments, though somewhat constricted in their descriptive power, also convey high dependency needs. Furthermore the comments convey resentment of other people and difficulty in relating to them. Clearly, afflicted spouses begin to restrict their social circle. The caregivers, however, convey a wish for widening their social contacts and a need to escape from the spousal relationship.

Three additional experiences, also exemplifying the caregiver's need to escape and the afflicted spouse's need to stay close to the spouse, were reported in this manner:

> He (afflicted spouse) just wants to sit in his chair and he wants me to sit on the couch. Then he is content. But I told him, "I can't; my mind is working good. If I stay in the house, we would both rot." So we take turns; for a while I let him have his way. Then I say, "We are going." If he doesn't come, I leave. But I worry about him, but I do go. The hardest thing is to leave. Once I went on a trip but got nothing out of it. What I was seeking for was what Jim and I had. But I can't find it. You can't run away from your problems; they are there when you get back.

Her husband merely said:

> I talk to the wife, no one else. What my trouble is, she will share it. . . . I let her have her way and go to her choice of restaurant.

Another caregiver said:

> I'm in limbo, I can't have another couple as friends, and I'm not a widow, so I can't join that crowd. I'm betwixt and between. . . . The biggest help is a neighbor that I have. She is a terrific friend. She takes care of us. I don't drive. She drives our car for us. I go to lunch with her and drag him along. He likes to get out. Mondays I go out when the girl (respite worker) is here, and then I do volunteer work at the hospital gift shop, though I had to give up some of it. I can talk with them, I love them, I go up there and get my laughs. And I escape by reading, close everything out and read, read.

Her husband had this to say about companionship:

> When friends come, I try to be civil. If they get on a subject like
> "you got a new red car and the neighbor has a red car, copy cat
> and all that," why get upset? Both paid the same. I try to change
> the subject if it's possible or excuse myself and walk out of the
> room.

And later he said:

> I talk to my wife. No, I'm not going to share with someone else and
> have them talk about it all over the place.

Again one can discern the afflicted spouse's need to restrict
his social circle; he cannot handle problems—even in conversa-
tions. In the next example, aloneness is poignantly expressed
by another caregiver wife:

> He follows me like a little kid. He walks a mile a minute. I told
> him, "I will put you in a nursing home," and he yelled, "Oh, no,
> hell, you won't." I have not mentioned it again. I feel I'm alone. I
> pray to the Lord to see me through and hope for better days. I
> haven't even been (Christmas) shopping this year. If I have him
> with me, you have to lead him everywhere.

And she added:

> I have very few people I can talk to. You can't explain to anyone if
> they haven't been through it. I talked to my nieces, and they were
> sympathetic, but what good does it do? None.

It is interesting to note that her husband expressed more
awareness of the situation than she seemed to indicate:

> She should go on a trip. Someone can stay with me. But she won't go.

Yet for some couples the caregiver did not voice the intense
need to get away but chose to stay close to the spouse. These
are their stories.

When I (caregiver spouse) go into another room or part of the home, he usually follows. I do not go out of the house, I do not leave him. He gets wild if he doesn't see me. I've given up my church group unless we can go together. I have worked profession-ally with patients and families. It gives me insight into my prob-lem. I don't work now because he becomes confused when he cannot find me. He is more important than I, so I take him with me. Every day I take him to the grocery store, the mall, or somebody's home to get him out. My friends are wonderful. They come by daily.

Her husband just said:

We do things together.

When illness occurs before the couple has reached retirement age and when the caregiver spouse has to work to provide an income, then "getting away" is not the pressing issue, but rather exhaustion and a painful realization of not being "normal." This is what a caregiver wife in her late 50s had to say:

We never do anything. There is not time to do anything—just work, eat, sleep, and go to church, and life is spent. I miss not being normal (crying). I already blocked that out. Now I know we are different, and I don't let myself miss it. It took me a long time to get where I am, to the acceptance stage, and I've come to the point where I appreciate what I have and have had in the past. I had a time when I resented it, all the financial mess we are in, his wrecking the car and losing his job. I thought it was his fault, but it wasn't his fault. I feel guilty for these thoughts, but I have them. I know he would do things for me and more. Not knowing what was wrong with him drove me crazy. If you know what you are dealing with, you can handle it better. Otherwise you have unre-alistic expectations.

Her husband, only recently diagnosed, still showed awareness of her needs:

We enjoy being with each other. We get to go to other places, which is good. She needs the interaction with the other ladies.

Most of the caregivers' answers came from wives because only six caregiver husbands were in this study. Some of the male caregivers' descriptions had a muted quality, although the same muted and accepting tone was present in some of the female caregivers. The following are examples:

> We clean the house together, and in the yard I let her hold things, like when I (caregiver husband) was cutting a piece of wood, I tell her what to hold. I'm happy as long as we are together; she is not demanding.

His afflicted wife said:

> We watch TV shows together. . . . I would like more time with him, but we have a good relationship, hope we always have it.

And later she said:

> I always talk to my husband. I don't really have close friends.

A caregiver wife who did not need to escape but who viewed the situation as a preparation for widowhood expressed it this way:

> Losing his companionship is hard, but he can still talk and go along with me. But when he gets frustrated, it upsets me. I know now what it is like to be lonely. It's a good preparation (for widowhood). I learned a lot.

Her husband said:

> We stay close together. I tell her anything; I have done that through all our married life.

This couple's example is particularly informative when relating it to Davis's (1985) speculation concerning relationships of *constant togetherness*. Davis hypothesized that feelings of loneliness will be fostered in the caregiver spouse and that such feelings may be a preparation for widowhood. The wife's comments quoted above seem to indicate that this indeed is happening.

Aloneness, sadness, and acknowledgment of the caregiver spouse's devotion also are expressed by the couple in the final example:

> We do little things together, but he doesn't remember them the next day. I (caregiver spouse) feel so sad about it. His oldest son has not talked to him for 2 years. He won't call or anything. Paul (husband) gets a strange look on his face when we talk about him (the son).

This is what her husband had to say about companionship and confiding in his wife:

> There is nothing to tell, nothing to worry about. I appreciate that she takes care of me. If I didn't have my present wife (this was his second marriage), I don't know where I would be; she's devoted to me.

Two major themes emerged from these reports: First, some caregiver spouses expressed a strong need to escape from the relationship, at least temporarily, while others were more accepting, almost content to be with the afflicted spouse. Second, some afflicted spouses had a need to "cling," or demand closeness; others appeared quiet and nondemanding. The two themes— the caregivers' need to escape and the afflicted spouses' clinging behavior—were tabulated to determine the frequency of such occurrences. Results are presented in Table 4.2.

The majority of caregiver spouses (63%) had a strong need to escape the relationship, and 37% were accepting or content to be at home with the spouse. Among afflicted spouses, 40% evidenced clinging or demanding behavior, but 60% did not.

The question arises whether an afflicted person's clinging and demanding behavior is associated with the other spouse's need to escape the relationship. A cross tabulation of the two variables was performed. Table 4.3 shows that when the afflicted spouse is not demanding and not clinging, the caregiver spouse's acceptance and the need to get away do not differ (30%

TABLE 4.2 Frequency of Dominant Themes: Caregiver and Afflicted Spouses

	n	%
Caregiver spouses (n = 30)		
Strong need to escape relationship	19	63
Accepting of, content with relationship	11	37
Total	30	100
Afflicted spouses (n = 30)		
Demanding, clinging	12	40
Low demand, not clinging	18	60
Total	30	100

in each situation). However, when the afflicted spouse is demanding and does cling, only 7% of the caregivers are accepting or content, and 33% need to escape the relationship, at least temporarily.

Although this trend was not statistically significant (because of the low frequency count in one of the cells), the effects of interactions on outcomes is demonstrated. The importance of including characteristics of the afflicted person's behavior in interactions with family caregivers is only beginning to be recognized in the literature (Deimling & Poulshock, 1985; McFall & Miller, 1990; Silliman & Sternberg, 1988).

TABLE 4.3 Cross Tabulation of Caregiver and Afflicted Spouses' Behavior

	Caregiver spouses					
	Accepting/ Content		Need to escape		Total	
	n	%	n	%	n	%
Afflicted spouses						
Not demanding, not clinging	9	30	9	30	18	60
Demanding, clinging	2	7	10	33	12	40
Total	11	37	19	63	30	100

SOURCE: From "The Impact of Alzheimer's Disease on the Marital Relationship" by L. K. Wright, 1991, *The Gerontologist, 31*(2), p. 232. Copyright © The Gerontological Society of America. Reprinted with permission.
NOTE: χ^2: 3.445, 1 df, $p < .063$; χ^2 with continuity correction: 2.159, 1 df, $p < .14$.

Well Couples

In sharp contrast to the loss of satisfying companionship among AD couples, well group couples reported much togetherness, they confided in each other, and they repeatedly stated how much they enjoyed each other's company. Four couples had a very close relationship and did practically everything together. They even commented that perhaps they "should not" be so close. Most couples, however, were willing to give each other "some space." Often their remarks described changes in their relationship brought about by retirement, but only a few couples had divergent interests leading to minor friction. Even then, the spouses were able to find solutions agreeable to both. When a spouse had some physical limitations affecting his or her outside interests, adaptation seemed uncomplicated and did not seem to impinge on the enjoyment of each other's companionship. Some typical cases are presented below.

Having all or most interests and activities together is expressed by these couples:

We walk together, we do church projects together, we exercise together, we go shopping together. We are together so much that if we are out alone, people ask, "Where is Lillian (other spouse)?" We like it to be that way.

And his wife commented:

We do most things together. Even on committees, it's always Lillian *and* Dave. But we know when to separate. We like to read. . . . When I have something that bothers me, I talk it over with Dave; we help each other. I may say to him, "Did I do the right thing?" And he may say, "Let's talk about it. Maybe you did, and maybe you didn't." He is a good listener. We are a unit. I don't go to other people for advice, but if I was single, I might need a confidant.

Obviously this couple has shared meaning in their communication patterns. They tell, they listen, they reflect, and they enjoy each other. Another husband described such sentiments succinctly when he said, "One of the pleasures we have is doing things together."

Pursuing many interests and activities together but separating occasionally are inherent in the next examples:

> We do many things together, but separately. Like at the club, the ladies do things together, and the men go off fishing. He will go hunting, and I'm (well wife) a director at our club, and I go on trips with the ladies. But if I have two activities in one week, he will remind me maybe not to get too involved. We are a couple first, but we allow each other time. We both work at our marriage. We try not to smother each other. . . . When I need to talk to someone, I talk to the Lord. I have tremendous faith. I don't even have a really close girlfriend I confide in. I talk to my husband. He is my confidant.

Her husband said the following:

> She belongs to different clubs, and I belong to different clubs; we have an understanding about that. We do things together, like going out with friends and to church. But separate activities are okay. I encourage it. She belongs to the garden club here in _____, and I helped her with a project recently.

Another well wife talked about how retirement affects companionship:

> When you are retired and together all day long, it's so different. It's good for him to go to the senior center and get away from me. It was different when we were working, we were not together all the time then. You should give each other space.

Her husband agreed in principle.

The following case shows that even friction over divergent interests does not destroy companionship:

> We (well husband and wife) are interested in each other, and we are considerate of each other's interests. We disagree on that occasionally but don't argue about it. Times apart are good; we give each other space but don't overdo it.

His wife stated it as follows:

TABLE 4.4 Major Types of the Companionship/Confidant
Dimension of Well Couples (*n* = 17 Couples)

	n	%
All, or almost all, activities and interests together	4	24
Some joint activities and interests:		
Allow "space":	7	41
Some discordance	4	24
Adapting of physical limitations	2	11
Total	17	100

> We have separate outside interests, but I will cancel mine and go
> with him, and he does the same. I rather do that.

Well couples in this study were relatively healthy people, although many were taking medications for some common health
problems, and some were experiencing physical limitations because of a heart condition or arthritis. Yet these limitations did not
seem to have the same negative impact on the relationship as the
cognitive impairment of the Alzheimer's afflicted person. One
wife from the well group talked about some adjustments she had
to make because of her husband's and her own health:

> Well, there are small things, like giving up my Sunday school class.
> That way, I didn't have to push him (to get up early). Or we avoid
> steps because of my arthritis.

Overall the theme for these couples is a synchronized life. A
frequency count of the slight variations in companionship is
presented in Table 4.4.

How Do Couples Cope
With Problems Pertaining to Companionship?

Well group spouses obviously communicate with each other,
and they are each other's close companion and ready confidant.
Taking the attitude of the other is the hallmark of their relation-

ships. However, when one spouse has Alzheimer's disease, many caregivers have a strong need to reach out to other people. Who is available for talking or for phone calls or who comes to visit and how much help caregiver spouses get that allows them time away from home are all related to coping with companionship issues. Before describing how couples in this study coped with companionship problems, some background information from other studies will be helpful.

Contact with and help from others is addressed often under the concept of *social support*. Shanas (1979) refuted the myths that older people in our mobile society have no or few contacts with children and other family members, but the issue has remained important in gerontological research. Interestingly, studies about the benefits of social support have not yielded entirely consistent results. In general, spouse caregivers report receiving fewer visits per month than daughters who are caregivers; those caregivers who receive more visits from family members and have stable social support seem to be less burdened, less stressed, and report the most positive mental health (Clipp & George, 1990; Lindgren, 1990; Zarit, Reever, & Bach-Peterson, 1980). However, several researchers found that neither informal social support (e.g., help from family members) nor formal social support (e.g., respite help) reduced the level of caregiver strain, burden, or depression (Gilleard, Gilleard, Gledhill, & Whittick, 1984; Robinson, 1989, 1990a). In another study the presence of more children and more use of services actually increased the risk of institutionalization for an afflicted spouse (Pruchno, Michaels, & Potashnik (1990). There is also some evidence that satisfaction with social support is more important to caregivers than the actual amount of support received (Clipp & George, 1990; Cutrona & Russell, 1987; Haley, Levine, Brown, & Bartolucci, 1987; Robinson, 1989; Tilden & Galyen, 1987).

To assess coping with companionship problems and related social support issues of couples in this study, spouses were asked (a) to report on the availability of support by naming persons or other sources of comfort, help, or information; (b) to report on the amount of informal support by counting the number of visits per month from family members, friends, and

TABLE 4.5 Current Sources of Comfort, Help, and Information: Frequencies of Sources Named by Caregiver, Afflicted, and Well Spouses*

	Caregiver spouses n = 30		Afflicted spouses n = 30		Well spouses n = 34	
	n	%	n	%	n	%
Family	30	100	14	47	32	94
Spouse primarily	—	—	16	53	13	38
Professionals	23	78	13	43	23	68
Friends, neighbors, colleagues	30	100	5	17	28	82
Aging agencies, ADRDA	15	50	—	—	1	3
Special TV programs or special topic readings	28	93	1	93	1	3
God, Bible**	3	10	—	—	2	6
No need	—	—	2	7	9	26
No one available	2	7	2	7	1	3
No specific answers	—	—	13	43	—	—

NOTE: *Respondents could name as many sources as they wished.
**God and the Bible were stated as primary sources of comfort, help, and information; however, in another context 81% of the respondents included prayer and trusting in God as important coping behavior.

neighbors; and (c) to report on the amount of formal support by counting the number of days per week that respite service was used (caregiver spouses only).

Availability of Support

Availability of other persons or resources was assessed by asking, "Who is the person you go to or talk to when you need comfort, help, or just information, and where else do you go for help?" Spouses could name as many persons or other sources as they wished. It is interesting to contrast answers from well group spouses, caregivers, and the afflicted spouses. These data are presented in Table 4.5.

Family members as source of comfort, help, and information were mentioned by all caregiver spouses and by 94% of the well spouses. Among afflicted spouses, 47% also named a family member and often specifically included a grandchild, but they named their own spouse even more often, 53% of the time. Their mates, however, did not name them once! This result poignantly demonstrates the loss of companionship for caregiver spouses.

Table 4.5 also shows that caregivers read everything they can find and watch every program about the illness; 93% in this sample reported doing so. In addition, caregivers use services geared to their needs, specifically the Alzheimer's and Related Disease Association (ADRDA). Support groups at these agencies play an important role in their lives. Only four caregiver spouses specifically stated that they did not want to attend such meetings. Their reasons ranged from not wanting to go unless there was a cure for the illness, to cost, to finding it too depressing, to considering support groups as a way of wallowing in self-pity.

One other interesting observation is that no caregiver spouse, but 26% of the well group spouses, felt no need to seek comfort or help or information. The well group spouses stated that they relied on themselves and that no one else could solve problems any better than they could. Two afflicted spouses apparently also had no need for help, but their reason was, "I don't have to," referring to perceiving their world as unproblematic.

Two caregivers and also one well group spouse specifically commented on changes in available support brought about by moving to a warmer climate and wanting to be closer to their children. The move, they stated, had been beneficial in some respects but also had brought loss of close friendships, and they had been unable to replace these friends. Two caregiver spouses stated that relating to a grown daughter under circumstances of illness was not easy because the daughter often had different ideas about "how Dad should be handled." Overall, however, other family members were seen as important sources of comfort, help, and information.

Amount of Informal Support:
Visits From Family, Friends, and Neighbors

Visits to the home from relatives, friends, and neighbors were assessed by asking couples to count the number of visits per month. If visits varied from month to month, an average based

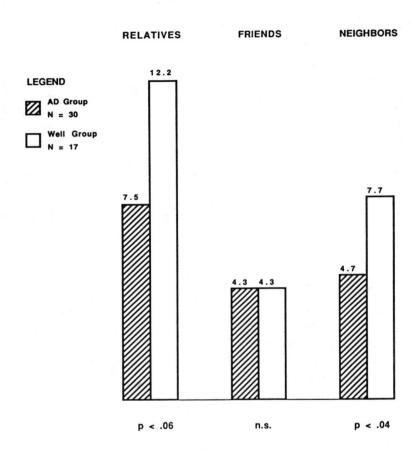

Figure 4.1. Average Number of Visits Per Month to the Home

on the past year's experience was estimated. A summary of these visits is presented in Figure 4.1.

Monthly visits from neighbors were significantly higher for well group couples than for AD group couples (8 for well versus 5 for AD group couples). Visits from relatives averaged 12 per month for well and 8 for AD group couples (this difference is only approaching statistical significance). Visits from friends were not significantly different for the two groups.

TABLE 4.6 Use of Day Care or Respite Care by Male and Female
              Caregivers

Days per week of day care or respite service	Male caregivers n = 6		Female caregivers n = 24	
	n	%	n	%
None	3	50	14	58
1 day/week	1	17	4	17
2 days/week	1	17	4	17
3 days/week	—	—	—	—
4 days/week	—	—	2	8
5 days/week	1	17	—	—
Total	6	100	24	100
Mean days/week		1.33		.833

NOTE: Percentages do not add to 100 due to rounding errors.
Mean number of days of services not significantly different for male and female spouses,
$p > .30$.

Eight monthly visits from relatives to AD couples is higher
than the average of five monthly visits to couples reported in
another study (Zarit et al., 1980). Nevertheless, when combining
all visits, AD couples in this study received considerably fewer
visits than well group couples—that is, approximately 16 visits
per month to AD couples versus an average of 24 visits per
month to well couples. Caregivers needed more, but they got
less. Clipp and George (1990) concluded that the caregivers'
need "does not necessarily elicit support" (p. S102), and Pruchno
(1990) concluded that informal help to spouse caregivers from
other family members is minimal.

Amount of Formal Support:
Respite Help and Day Care

The amount of respite help used by caregiver spouses was assessed by asking how many days per week they had either a respite
worker come to the home or used a day-care center for the afflicted
spouse. The two types of services were combined. A comparison of
service use by husband and wife caregivers is presented in Table 4.6.

A surprising finding is that the majority of caregivers did
not use any services: 50% of the husband and 58% of the wife

caregivers were without formal support. This low use of formal services is consistent with other reports (George, Fillenbaum, & Burchett, 1988; Lawton, Brody, & Saperstein, 1989; Montgomery & Borgatta, 1989). The husbands in this study used services more often than did the wives, but the difference is not statistically significant. In addition, there seemed to be equal concern by husbands and wives for the quality of the services provided. One male caregiver whose wife had attended a day-care center reported that he pulled her out for the following reasons: The room in which the day-care program was being held was too small, there was an odor in the room, only one bathroom was available, the other afflicted persons were all black, and he felt they were in worse conditions than his wife. He instead had a respite worker come to the home one day per week, which allowed him to get away alone. Similarly a female caregiver who also decided against a day-care program reported that she evaluated a particular day-care center by participating in the program for a whole day as if she were the patient! "It was awful," she said. "By the end of the day, they were crying and so agitated; I wouldn't want my husband to be in that situation. Maybe I will need to do it when he gets worse, but not now." She also had a respite worker come to her home once a week. The use of respite workers, however, presented problems for some wife caregivers. Two specifically mentioned that no male respite workers are available and that they did not feel comfortable leaving the husband alone at home with a female respite worker.

Overall it appears that husbands and wives do not differ greatly in their use of outside services, and caregivers identified several barriers to this type of coping. It is interesting to note that Quayhagen and Quayhagen (1988) found the use of respite time to have little if any association with well-being for wife caregivers, and it had a negative association with well-being for husband caregivers. The authors posited feelings of guilt when care is turned over to someone else as a possible explanation of their findings. In light of this study, however, use of respite time needs to take the afflicted person's behavior into consideration; the caregivers' need for services will be great when they have to cope with clinging, demanding, and other difficult behaviors. Perhaps equally important in determining use and benefits of services is the quality of available services.

HUMAN DEVELOPMENT
AND MARITAL COMPANIONSHIP

Two people who interact with each other will change each other. Companionship within a marital relationship epitomizes interactions and demonstrates that interactions are essential for human development. However, memory problems in one spouse affect interactions and mutual companionship. For AD couples, therefore, asynchronized biological, psychological, and sociocultural life dimensions can be expected with corresponding outcomes of control or disorder and adaptation or distortion. Well couples, too, could experience problems over companionship and hence asynchronized psychological and sociocultural life dimensions with resulting outcomes of concordance or discordance and acculturation or exploitation (Riegel, 1976; see Table 1.1).

Findings from this study show that marital companionship for well group couples leads to synchronized life dimensions: The overwhelming majority evidence enjoyment of each other's company. A few couples recognize that their relationship is perhaps "too close," an indication of some projection to eventual widowhood and awareness that loss of such closeness might bring problems. Most well group couples, however, allow each other "some space." Hence there is little evidence of one partner exploiting the other. On a few occasions, some minor adaptation because of a spouse's physical limitations is necessary.

For AD couples the data presented in this chapter provide evidence of different outcomes when—because of cognitive impairment—the inner-biological, the psychological, and the sociocultural dimensions of development are not synchronized. A poignant example of attempts at adaptation but resulting distortions is the account given by an early stage male afflicted spouse who used to love playing golf. He still tries to relate to others, but memory problems lead to counting the wrong score, and it affects relationships with his friends. Their tolerance of him (after he told them of his problem) is interpreted as "Maybe I am getting better." But the fact that most of the time he refuses to play the game he once loved shows that he is aware of his diminished ability to interact with others. He therefore narrows his circle to that of his wife's companionship alone.

The same afflicted spouse, when asked whom he would go to for comfort and help, replied: "My wife, all the time. . . . There's no place to go. I felt with the neurologist, they put me off. I got that feeling at (the university clinic); I wanted to ask questions, but they weren't about to help me."

This early stage Alzheimer's victim not only is suffering from his own memory loss but also is pushed farther into isolation by other people's perceptions of him. He is, to state it in Meadian theory, quite accurately aware of other people's definitions of the situation and of the gestures made by them toward him (Mead, 1977; Thomas, 1923). Yet it is his own gestures (or behaviors), his constricted activity and perseveration in communication, that contribute to other people's evaluations of him. His behaviors are, in part, the result of his illness, and thus he becomes unable to control other people's actions. His own behaviors lack shared meaning with those of well people. He is therefore "irrational" (Mead, 1934, p. 334) or is perceived as "senile" (Chappell & Orbach, 1986).

Beisecker, Wright, and Kasal (1991) reported that many physicians ignore the AD patient during office visits, and as the disease progresses, physicians increasingly communicate with family caregivers only. Yet as this study shows, many early to middle stage afflicted persons are still aware of their own behaviors; in fact, 27% of afflicted spouses in this study showed such awareness. Although the disease process may not be altered by talking with afflicted persons, their sense of isolation can. They are human beings with their own social world, not just patients with a diagnosis of Alzheimer's disease.

In contrast to the constricted life dimensions of afflicted spouses, human development for the caregiver spouses is quite remarkable. They attempt to control a part of their lives by seeking other companionship. Their comments evidence acceptance and adaptation and wisdom derived from prolonged inner struggle. Two of the most poignant descriptions were given by caregiver wives. One had tried to find a new relationship (with another man), but, as she put it, "What I was seeking for was what Jim and I had. But I can't find it. You can't run away from your problems; they are there when you get back."

The other caregiver recounted the difficult time prior to knowing that her husband's troublesome behaviors were due to an illness. "It took me a long time to get where I am, to the acceptance stage," she said, "and I've come to the point where I appreciate what I have and have had in the past." She was confident that, had she been ill, her husband would have cared for her: "He would do things for me and more." These caregivers' adaptation is a triumph in human development.

In summary, findings about the companionship dimension of marriage for the two groups can be contrasted by describing well couples as two people moving together in harmony, while AD couples are two people living together, each in different worlds of awareness yet unable to leave the relationship. The afflicted spouses adapt by increased dependency in order to prevent total disorder, and their mates adapt by accepting a caregiver role or by seeking other forms of companionship. The difference between these two groups of couples is indeed significant.

ASSESSMENT STRATEGIES AND INTERVENTION GUIDELINES

In light of the above findings and other research reports, the following assessment strategies and intervention guidelines for companionship issues are offered.

Assessment Strategies

Health professionals can assess a couple's companionship by addressing four issues: (a) How often do couples engage in mutual activities? (b) Do caregivers have a need for other companionship?

(c) How much informal and how much formal support is available? (d) How satisfied is the caregiver with available support? For assessing how often couples engage in mutual activities, the companionship (cohesion) subscale of Spanier and Thompson's (1982) Dyadic Adjustment Rating Scale can be used (items of this subscale and scoring methods are described at the beginning of this chapter). The scale items are also useful for asking spouses to comment on the quality of their companionship and for assessing whether they have needs for other companions. As one caregiver spouse said during the interview, "You know, filling out that form made me realize where I'm at," meaning that the questions on the scale helped her evaluate her own situation. Many caregivers, therefore, can use these assessment strategies themselves to gain a better understanding of "where they are at."

It is also important to question afflicted spouses. In fact, companionship issues will elicit more comments than any other questions. Patience, very careful listening, and note taking rather than tape recordings are advised because afflicted spouses tend to dislike recorders. It is worth the effort to assess an afflicted spouse's level of awareness or level of distortion pertaining to interactions with the caregiver; it provides rich data for interventions that can be discussed with the caregiver spouse.

To assess informal support, caregivers can be asked to estimate, on average, how often family members, friends, and neighbors visit their homes. Some caregivers can easily give a monthly average; others may need to think about periods of 6 months or an entire year because some out-of-town relatives visit infrequently. An average per month still can be calculated.

To assess formal support, the use of respite services to the home or the use of day-care centers can be questioned. Perceived quality of support is an additional but crucial assessment component and must be questioned for all available support.

Intervention Guidelines

Intervention implies that some specific situation requires change. Relatively healthy older couples might not perceive a need for change, although a few couples in this study wondered whether they perhaps were "too close." Clinicians, therefore, should encourage involvement in outside activities. Accounts from same-age peers and the companionship patterns listed in Table 4.4 can serve as useful catalysts for discussions. For AD couples, frequency and quality of day-to-day interactions will be the focus of interventions. First, it is important to emphasize that frequent interactions between caregiver and afflicted spouses are important; interactions reassure the afflicted spouse, reduce fears of abandonment, and even may reduce clinging and demanding behaviors (Beck & Heacock, 1988; Hall, 1988). Caregiver spouses, husbands and wives alike, are remarkable in their patience and ingenuity for structuring interactions. They need encouragement to adapt interactions to the ability level of the afflicted spouse. For example, instead of discussing political events, they could talk about the grandchildren's school activities, pictures in a magazine, the color of plants. "Doing things together" may be as simple as asking the afflicted spouse to hold a piece of wood (as one caregiver husband in this study did), or doing a jigsaw puzzle together, going for a walk together, or watching TV together. The many household tasks described in Chapter 2 are also ways of interacting with the spouse. The important principle to convey to caregivers is that they do not need to eliminate joint activities—they only have to "modify them to a simpler form" (Hall, 1988, p. 40).

But all of these efforts demand energy from the caregiver, and, if in addition the afflicted spouse is very demanding and clings to the spouse at every step, the caregiver's need for other companionship becomes a priority for intervention (Gwyther & Matteson, 1983). Caregivers may recognize their own needs but still may be reluctant to seek help; they may think that it is better to wait with looking for help until the very late stages of the illness or when the spouse becomes incontinent. If this is the caregiver's perception, then health professionals must give caregivers not only practical assistance with obtaining help but also psychological support; caregivers need to get away without feeling guilty. It can be pointed out that some afflicted spouses are aware of their mates' need for other companionship. Caregivers can be reassured that regular, early help is actually better: The helper will get to know the afflicted spouse's likes and dislikes, as well as troublesome behaviors, and the helper can become a familiar face to him or her and thus provide social stability (Roberts & Algase, 1988). If a familiar person stays, clinging to the caregiver spouse actually may be reduced, and the caregiver can leave without it causing problems. How the "free" time is spent is the caregivers' choice. Caregivers who are unfamiliar with support groups may be encouraged to attend such meetings, where many practical issues of care are discussed. Although most caregivers find support groups very helpful and a source of strength, they have the right to choose their own social contacts.

Assessing how much informal and formal support is already available to the caregiver is therefore important information for planning interventions. It seems that, in general, AD couples get fewer visits from family members and friends than well couples, but why people curtail visits is not really known. Perhaps feelings of vulnerability ("Could I be like this one day?") and helplessness of not knowing "what to say" or "what to do" are underlying causes. If informal support is low, Robinson (1988) advocated that health professionals intervene by arranging a joint meeting between the primary caregiver and members of his or her entire natural social network, including family members, neighbors, and friends. How to provide assistance to the caregiver and problems associated with helping are discussed openly during such meetings. The health professional becomes the leader and facilitator of such sessions so that members of the network themselves engage in problem solving. It should be noted that this intervention, which has been termed *network therapy* (Garrison & Howe, 1976), requires the health professional to have skills in conducting group therapy.

Network therapy can be successful, but health professionals also will encounter long-standing family problems that cannot be resolved in one or two meetings. Caregivers, therefore, need to be supported in seeking out those family members and friends who are easy to be with and avoiding those who bring conflicts or arguments over how the afflicted person should be cared for.

In other words, the caregiver's satisfaction with support is crucial. Health professionals also need to assess whether assertive social skills are lacking and whether caregivers need to be taught how to ask for help (Robinson, 1990b). For example, asking specifically, "Can you stay with your dad on Saturday from 2 p.m. to 6 p.m.?" will get a definite response; but sighing and hinting for help with, "You have no idea what it is like not to be able to get away" is less likely to get the desired help. When family members or friends come to stay with the afflicted person and the caregiver can get away, caregivers can be encouraged to offer something in return. This reciprocity keeps relationships balanced, and caregivers will feel more comfortable about asking for help again (Cutrona & Russell, 1987; Tilden & Galyen, 1987). For example, caregivers can offer to pick up the dry cleaning on the way home, to hem a skirt, or to mend some equipment.

Formal support can consist of hired respite help (someone comes to the couple's home) or organized day-care programs (outside the couple's home). Financial barriers to obtaining such help need to be discussed, and caregivers need to be told about programs for which fees for services are based on a sliding scale. The caregiver's trust in the respite worker again touches on satisfaction with support, and helping caregivers find what is acceptable to them is the health professional's responsibility. The caregiver should interview the prospective respite worker, ask about previous experiences, obtain references, and, once an acceptable person has been found, make plans for familiarizing the respite worker with the afflicted spouse's behaviors. The caregiver initially can stay within easy physical reach (stay in another room or be outside) until he or she feels comfortable with the respite worker's ability to handle different situations.

Day-care centers are the other type of formal social support. In this study, caregivers as well as afflicted spouses mentioned not only concerns over the physical environment of such places but also racial issues. "They are all black there," said one afflicted spouse when he refused to go to the day-care center. This issue rarely is acknowledged in the gerontological literature. But these older persons grew up during a time when segregation was the cultural norm. Thus an afflicted spouse's comments more likely reflect the remembered past rather than any racial bias per se. This issue may become less important as the present middle-aged generation becomes the older generation of tomorrow.

Over the last 5 years, the number of available day-care programs has grown, and many now have trained staff members and offer structured activities specifically designed for cognitively impaired persons (Baldwin, 1990). Nevertheless caregivers are to be encouraged to visit programs before they enroll a spouse, and day-care staff need to ask caregivers about troublesome behaviors that may require special approaches. Identified troublesome behaviors should not be used for screening out clients; rather, the caregiver's experiences need to be incorporated into the plan of care to be used during the day. In addition, directors of day-care centers need to ask caregivers to evaluate their programs periodically. Such evaluations could be done anonymously to guarantee honest responses.

Finally clinicians need to ask caregivers to "stand back" and evaluate for themselves how satisfied they are with the help they are getting. If they are not satisfied, they need to realize that this is one aspect of their lives over which they can have control. How much help they get and who helps them can be changed to meet their needs.

FIVE

Affection and Sexuality Within the Marital Relationship

INTRODUCTION

Emotional and physical attractions, as well as affectional gestures and physical intimacy between spouses, are part of a happy marriage relationship. Several researchers have found that older couples in the general population report an increase in emotional closeness (Reedy, Birren, & Schaie, 1982) and a decrease in sexual intimacy over the course of marriage (Brubaker, 1985; Starr, 1985; Walz & Blum, 1987). But information on this sensitive subject pertaining to spouses in caregiver-care receiver relationships is sparse.

EXPLORING AFFECTION AND SEXUALITY

Issues pertaining to affection and sexuality were explored with three major questions: (a) How much affection and sexual intimacy do couples report? (b) How much do both groups of couples agree over affection and sexual intimacy, and are husbands and wives similar or different in their assessment of agreement? and (c) What problems are encountered, and how do couples cope with issues pertaining to affection and sexuality?

How Much Affection and Sexual Intimacy Do Couples Report?

Spouses were interviewed separately for both the affection and sexuality questions. To assess type and frequency of affectional gestures between spouses, the affection subscale of the Dyadic Adjustment Rating Scale was revised on the basis of Spanier and Thompson's (1982) suggestion that more items measuring affection need to be added to this scale. The new subscale included the original item "kissing the spouse" and five additional indicators: "touching the spouse lovingly," "caressing the spouse," "holding hands," "putting an arm around the spouse," and "sleeping in the same bed." The response options for the new items were the same as for the original "kissing the spouse," ranging from *every day* (5) to *never* (1). The maximum score, representing high affection, was 30; a score of 6 indicated no affection.

The average number of affectional gestures was 21 for AD group couples and 25 for well group couples. The scores seem to indicate fairly high affection for both groups. But averaged scores are misleading: Some couples reported no or very low affection on the affection scale, while others indicated very high affection.

Sexual intimacy was assessed by asking each spouse to report frequency of sexual intercourse per month. Eight afflicted spouses gave answers different from those of the respective caregiver spouse. Six of these eight afflicted spouses claimed they were sexually active when, according to the caregiver spouse, they were not. The afflicted spouses' answers were considered to be less accurate. Therefore the comparison between the AD and well group couples that follows uses only the caregiver spouses' answers for the AD group. Well group spouses gave practically identical answers; however, only one spouse's answer from each well group couple was chosen for the comparison analysis. (Details

TABLE 5.1 Reported Sexual Intimacy per Month: Alzheimer's Versus Well Couples

Intimacy level	AD couples		Well couples	
	n	%	n	%
No activity	19	63	2	12
Occasional tries, attempts, snuggles	3	10	1	6
Sexual intimacy (monthly)				
< 1	—	—	2	12
1-2	1(F)[a]	3	3	17
2	—	—	1	6
3-4	2(F)[a]	7	3	17
4-5	—	—	1	6
6-8	1[b]	3	2[c]	12
10	2[b]	7	2[b]	12
14	2[b]	7	—	—
Subtotal of sexually active couples	8	27	14	82
Mean (all ages)	8		3.8*	
Mean (ages > 60)	7.2		2.4*	
Total	30	100	17	100

SOURCE: From "The Impact of Alzheimer's Disease on the Marital Relationship" by L. K. Wright, 1991, *The Gerontologist, 31*(2), p. 230. Copyright © The Gerontological Society of America. Reprinted with permission.
NOTE: a. F = couples with female afflicted spouses.
b. One couple both spouses < 60 years old.
c. Two couples both spouses < 60 years old.
*$p < .004$.

of this method of analysis can be found in the Appendix under "Data Analysis With Quantified Scales").

No sexual activity was reported by 63% of AD group couples but by only 12% of well group couples. In addition, 10% of AD and 6% of well group couples reported "occasional tries, attempts, snuggles," to use their own words. Regular sexual intimacy per month was reported by 82% of well and 27% of AD group couples, and frequency of contacts also differed for the two groups. Contacts ranged from 1-2, 3-4, 6-8, 10, or 14 and more times per month for AD couples. Well group couples reported sexual contacts ranging from fewer than once per month to 10 times per month. As shown in Table 5.1, none of the well group couples reported sexual intercourse to be more than 10 times per month.

When excluding "occasional tries, attempts, snuggles" and comparing only the sexually active couples, sexual intimacy took place twice as often between couples in the AD group as between couples in the well group: approximately 8 per month for the AD group, and approximately 4 per month for the well group. In each group, however, three couples were age 60 or below. Because age is a definite factor in frequency of sexual intercourse, the six couples were excluded from the analysis; this exclusion resulted in an average frequency of 2.4 per month for the well group and 7.2 for the AD group. The difference is statistically significant.

The much higher average in the AD group reflects high sexual activity of 10 and 14 or more times per month initiated or demanded by male afflicted spouses. Couples with a female afflicted spouse did not report such high frequencies. High sexual activity occurred among 14% of all AD group couples; but when the nonsexually active couples are excluded from the analysis, high sexual activity occurred among 50% of sexually active AD group couples.

How Much Agreement Over Affection and Sexual Intimacy Do Couples Report?

Not only frequency of sexual contacts was assessed but also agreement over affection and sexuality. Spouses were asked whether they always or never agreed on affection and sexual issues, on showing love, or on being too tired for sex. The maximum agreement scores for affection and sexuality were 9, the lowest were 2. A summary of agreement scores is presented in Table 5.2.

No significant differences between spousal dyads from both groups were noted over issues of affection. Agreement over sexual issues, however, showed that male afflicted spouses gave significantly higher agreement ratings than their female caregiver spouses. The couples' statements given in the next section will explain why.

TABLE 5.2 Mean Agreement Over Affection and Sexuality Scores by Group and Couple Comparison

	Group comparison (means)		
	Alzheimer's group		*Well group*
	n = 30		n = 17
1. Affection	7.4		7.9
2. Sexuality	6.7		7.8

		Couple comparison (means)			
Female caregiver	*Male AD*	*Male caregiver*	*Female AD*	*Female*	*Male*
n = 24	n = 24	n = 6	n = 6	n = 17	n = 17
1. 7.3	8.0	7.5	7.8	7.8	7.9
2. 6.7	8.0*	6.7	8.3	7.4	7.7

NOTE: 1. Agreement over affection: Possible range of scores: 9 = high, 2 = low. 2. Agreement over sexuality: Possible range of scores: 9 = high, 2 = low.
*$p < .01$.

Reported Problems and Coping With Issues Pertaining to Affection and Sexuality

Problems and coping themes related to affectional and sexual issues were assessed by asking spouses to elaborate on answers they had given on the previously described quantitated measures. The responses from both group of couples will be presented and summarized in Table 5.3 for the AD group and Table 5.4 for the well group.

AD Couples

The AD couples' answers were so diverse that it was difficult to discern a pattern. Some caregiver spouses were very affectionate toward the afflicted spouse whether or not sexual intimacy occurred. Others rejected both affection and sexuality, and the afflicted spouse seemed to be quite aware of this. Some caregivers were affectionate but abstained sexually; others sought new relationships. Several caregivers with a male afflicted spouse reported clinging, childlike type of affection and attempts at or demands for frequent sexual contacts. Some typical examples follow.

The first example represents a situation with no or rare affection and no sexual activity. The male caregiver said the following:

> She doesn't want hugging; it started about 4 years ago. I don't force myself on her; it saves a lot of arguments that way. It doesn't bother me, I'm too old for that anyway. That's the thing about growing old.

His wife, when questioned about being affectionate or being intimate, replied:

> Not for years. . . . I just stand by, do nothing.

She also said that she was "extremely unhappy" in her marriage, a statement that her husband attributed to her illness. Although there was no expression of tenderness between them, he did care for her physical needs in a determined manner.

In the next example, the caregiver wife was very loving and accepting. She said:

> There is no sex. He can't get it up. It doesn't bother me, but it bothers him; he's ashamed to admit it. It's his male ego. He is so shy. We are always affectionate, we both are. He's the sweetest man I've ever known. He has never spoken a cross word to me. . . . No, I would never look for someone else. None would come up to this one.

Her husband seemed embarrassed when questioned about affection and sexual relations. He laughed and said:

> Not often, maybe once a month.

In the following case the afflicted spouse acknowledged his frustration. His wife's comments will be noted first:

> He talks about his impotence, and when he sees articles, he asks to go to meetings where they discuss it, but I can't drive with my heart condition, it's not a good idea. It never bothered me. It was kind of a relief. I felt rejected for a while but knew I wasn't really. We didn't talk about it. He just made silly remarks. We still give each other hugs and rubbing the back, we still do it.

Her husband, at times tangential and at times mumbling incomprehensibly, gave these answers:

> The worst problem . . . I am getting older. . . . When it (impotence) smacks you in the face, what else would you think about? Those ads (advertisements), they say it can be reversed. . . . Believe it if I see it? . . . Miss it? . . . (laughs) . . . But what in the hell can I do about it? That's what bugs me about the question.

He was right, of course; the interviewer's questions could not help him. His wife had accurately assessed his mood, and although she showed her affection with hugging and rubbing his back, she was reluctant to ease his sexual frustrations.

In the next case, however, the caregiver wife seems reluctant about showing affection and voices outright rejection and even a hint of disgust for a sexual relationship with an afflicted spouse. She said:

> I think he has more affection for me than I have for him. That's when he knows me, and most times he does. Sometimes we hug, but there is no sex now. He stopped years ago. That's all right with me that he showed no interest. I don't' miss it. You don't *want* a relationship with someone like *that*.

The couple's past marital relationship had not been happy; in fact, she had contemplated divorce just prior to her husband being diagnosed with probable Alzheimer's disease. She sheltered and provided for him, but she could not love him. Excerpts from her husband's comments are revealing:

> She doesn't like that (putting an arm around her), thinks I have something else in mind. She doesn't like to be fondled. I don't argue about it. I just accept it. Why argue? After all, she is very important around here. . . . It's a long time ago (having sex). You outgrow it. It wasn't the easiest to accept. Dummy me (slaps his forehead with his hand), you force yourself on her. I try to be considerate, saves a lot of arguments that way.

This afflicted spouse was quite aware of his wife's rejection, and his comment "after all, she is very important around here" may be his way of saying that she is in control of the situation. His awareness of her feelings restricted his gestures and actions.

How intertwined memory and intimacy are is epitomized in the following case. The caregiver husband said:

> She is affectionate but has no memory. We touch and hold hands and embrace, yes, but no sex for over a year. She wouldn't reject me, but she wouldn't remember from one moment to the next. So I just abstain. I just deal with it. I'm getting to the age where it's not as bad as 4 or 5 years ago. We had lots of good years, 35 of them. You can't forget all that.

There was sadness in his voice. He obviously loved his wife, and although she too quite emphatically said, "I love him," he did not want to exploit her. Not being able to share memories of and during intimacy would have been too painful for him, and so he "just abstained."

Some caregivers showed little affection but still expressed interest in sexual matters. Remarks about building or seeking other relationships were included in their comments. A caregiver wife said the following:

> After you find out you can't have sex anymore, you either forget it or get it somewhere else. Once in a while my body calls out for it. Maybe it's still in his head, but it's not in his hands. He makes no more advances; there's no intimacy, no show of affection. Two years ago he had an implant, but it didn't help. . . . At one time I felt I needed someone, but I never have, and I hope I won't. You can't go against good years. I would not run out on him now, I promised. But thoughts have been there, though I fought myself against it, and I've always won. The want is there, the nerve is not.

Her husband gave a totally different evaluation of their relationship:

> We have lots of affection. (And about sexual activity) No problems there, 3 or 4 times per week.

Perhaps it was "still in his head," as his wife had pondered, but it did not help her in her restlessness.

Compensating for lack of affection and sexuality is shown with the next answers given by a male caregiver:

> It's been 19 years since I had sex with my wife. That disagreement started shortly after we were married. She had no interest. Yes, I do miss it; I'm not completely unfunctional. I use VCRs and fantasy as a substitute, but it isn't satisfying; the emotional is missing. You want to give pleasure to her. You can masturbate all you want, but it isn't the same. . . . I have someone (a woman friend), we can talk together, but it's not a physical relationship at this time.

His wife's answers were constricted. About being affectionate she said:

> Very seldom now, like most old people. It doesn't trouble me . . . (pause). I did not have an average childhood; I learned to be tough.

Her husband obviously was not ready to define himself "like most old people," yet it seemed as if she wanted to give an explanation or apology for the present situation.

The gradual worsening of the relationship is represented with the next case. The female caregiver said:

> There's nothing now, and there is no way to compensate for it, just love from the grandchildren, but it's not the same. Some people just aren't very affectionate. I've accepted that a long time ago. He's been impotent for 8 years; it gradually got worse, but acknowledging it is another thing. I wanted him to go to the doctor and tell him, but he said, "No, no." He bothered me constantly, sexually, he was so frustrated, and I have chronic cystitis, that's a problem. Now his doctor has put him on Mellaril (a major tranquilizer), and now there's nothing. Sometimes I would just like to hug him, but I'm afraid it will bring back all that sexual stuff.

The afflicted husband showed awareness of his wife's feelings but also indicated that he had not lost interest in sexual matters:

> It's this condition. Oh, yes, I'm interested, at least once a week. But . . . (hostility in his voice) she don't want these hands on her. (And about being affectionate) Depends on how she is treating me.

Frequent or even hypersexual activity was reported in several cases. One caregiver wife explained it this way:

If he gets upset, I hug him and kiss him and it seems to have a calming effect on him. But intimate sex, it's harder for him than it used to be, and it can't be as often, and that bothers him. Now it's not a problem for me because I've never been highly sexual anyway, but I've always tried to satisfy his needs, and I still do. He can't get an erection as often, sometimes he loses it before he can climax, and that's a problem for him. Naturally it's a little bit of a problem for me. I mean, after two or three times, naturally, it gets on my nerves, but I try to let him know . . . (pause). I know he still has his desires, but you just can't. We used to have sex at least every other day, and then it became every 3 or 4 days. But he says the longer he goes, the harder it is for him, and he gets frustrated.

Her husband showed some awareness of his wife's feelings:

Oh, yes, we are intimate 3 or 4 times a week. I make an appointment with her, but if she is tired, I try not to bother her.

Different needs, different emotions, resentment and frustration—yet each spouse was trying to accommodate as well as influence the other's actions.

Some resentment is also apparent in this wife caregiver's report:

He tells me a hundred times a day how much he loves me, and I tell him, too, that I love him. He would have sex every day if I was able to accommodate him. But I noticed his erections are less strong than in the past. For a while he was on medications and could not get an erection at all, and I had to be the initiator. I resented that.

Her husband, when questioned about sexual activity, said:

Never too tired. We enjoy it; three times a week this last year or a little less.

His answer would indicate that he was unaware of his wife's resentment. Yet this same afflicted spouse had voiced understanding and concerns for his wife's need to have friends and companionship outside the home.

Well Couples

The well couples' descriptions of affection and sexuality do not indicate the interpersonal drama evident in the AD couples' relationships. Only two dominant types of relationships emerged: (a) moderate to high levels of affectional expression with infrequent sexual intimacy and (b) various levels of affection with regular sexual activity. Two other situations, rare affection without sexual interest and low affection with some verbal expression of sexual interest, were reported by only one couple in each category. Examples of these latter two situations will be presented first.

> (husband) Affection? It's adequate for both of us. We have been married so long plus 6 years of dating first. . . . There is no sex now, not since 6 to 8 years ago.

His wife explained their relationship as follows:

> I am not real affectionate. He is kind of more affectionate, but we seem to get along all right. Most couples today expect the physical act to continue, but it's downhill with age; the spiritual and emotional is going up. We both have grown to a point where the physical is not important anymore because the physical goes . . . with his heart trouble and his hernia and all. But we have been satisfied with other things, like being congenial. I have not missed it.

The relationship of the next couple was not limited by the husband's but rather by the wife's physical (arthritic) condition.

> (wife) Being intimate stopped 2 years ago because intercourse was hurting, and even touching was hurting. I went to the doctor, but the medicine did not seem to help. We would probably be closer if we still had sex, but who knows? We have single beds, but sometimes we lie on the same bed together.

Her husband also attributed the situation to advancing age, but some disappointment resonated in his words:

We are winding down with age. I could do it, but she does not want to. It doesn't frustrate me. Would be nice, but . . .

Infrequent sexual intimacy was reported by three couples and was attributed mainly to the husband's ability to perform. As one male spouse described it:

We have not had sex for 2 months now because of my (prostate) problem. It doesn't create a problem, not that I know of.

His wife said:

We usually hug each other in the morning and before going to bed and sometimes during the day. I would say we are about the same in expressing affection. But sex? Very occasionally now, two or three times per year. He seems to have a hard time having an erection. Our sex life used to be very good, and I'm always willing. But it's not really a problem. He is very affectionate otherwise.

Most well couples, however, reported regular, mutually satisfying sexual intimacy, and only one spouse stated that his "sexual appetite" was greater than his wife's. Well couples seemed more concerned over who was or was not expressing enough affection rather than over differences in sexual interest. The following is a typical example:

I think she is more aggressive in terms of affection than I. That's probably so with most women now, different than 40 years ago. I like it though (laughs). She will kiss me on top of the head, little things like that, and I reach up so she can reach me. We still have a good sex life, enjoy it as much as ever.

It was amusing to hear his wife trying to guess what he had told the interviewer about affection:

He would say that he is more affectionate, but I say I am more affectionate. Sexually, oh (pause), about every 10 days, but not if it's cold.

Summary of Types of Relationships

The couples' reports are summarized in Table 5.3 for the AD group and in Table 5.4 for the well group. Because of the wide range in amount of affection and different patterns in sexuality, it was difficult to categorize the relationships. Nevertheless seven categories of relationship patterns could be discerned for the AD group, but only four of these patterns applied to the well group. Each category identifies whether affection was high or low and how much sexual activity occurred. Coping themes corresponding to these categories were derived from the spouses' answers; they are listed in adjacent columns in Tables 5.3 and 5.4, respectively. In the last column, an interpretation of developmental outcomes resulting from the couples' interactions is given; outcomes will be discussed under the section entitled "Human Development Related to Affection and Sexuality."

AD Group

Some general observations can be made about the relationship patterns of the AD group. It appears that varying degrees of affection and absence of sexual intimacy were acceptable to most spouses because they considered themselves "too old for that anyhow" (Categories I and II, Table 5.3).

When affection is absent or very low and there is only verbal, not actual, expression of sexual interests (Category III), then caregivers are more likely to attempt other relationships. Two caregivers (one male, one female) were seeking new (opposite-sex) relationships, but neither contemplated a divorce. The respective afflicted spouses seemed unaware of their mates' feelings and sexual longings and distorted the situation: Both claimed they were still sexually active, the female spouse claiming "very seldom now" and the male spouse claiming "three or four times per week." Yet another afflicted spouse in Category III was aware of his situation. Both he and his caregiver wife still expressed sexual interest verbally. He claimed they were still sexually active "at least once a week," but she controlled (had eliminated) his excessive sexual demands through medications. This caregiver was

TABLE 5.3 Affection, Sexual Intimacy, Coping Themes, and Developmental Outcomes for Couples in the Presence of Alzheimer's Disease ($n = 30$)

Category/Relationship characterization	Coping Themes		Developmental Outcomes Caregiver-Afflicted	% couples
	Caregiver (n)	Afflicted (n)		
I. No or rare affection, no sexual interest	Too old; don't want to be bothered (3)	Too old; sex is bothersome (3)	Concordance	10
	Too old (1)	Unhappy (1F)	Discordance	3
II. Moderate to high affection, no sexual interest	Too old; never sexy (2)	Too old (1)	Concordance	3
		Doesn't trouble me (1)	Concordance	3
III. No or rare affection, verbal expression of sexual interest	Attempt at other relationships; VCR; masturbation (2)	No problem and distorts frequency (1)	Adaptation and distortion	3
		Too old and distorts frequency (1F)	Adaptation and distortion	3
	Afraid of sex; medication control (1)	Hostility; verbal demands and distorts frequency (1)	Discordance and distortion (control and disorder)	3
IV. Moderate to high affection, verbal expression of sexual interest	Minimize as just one part of life (3)	Very affectionate (2)	Adaptation and concordance	7
		My fault; distorts meaning for spouse (1)		
	Abstain (1)	Very affectionate (1F)	Adaptation and distortion	3
	It's a relief (1)	What can I do about it? (1)	Adaptation and concordance	3
	Love and accept (1)	Distorts frequency (1)	Distortion and adaptation	3
	Frustration (2)	Distorts frequency (2)	Adaptation and distortion	3
	Frustration (1)	No answer (1)	Discordance and distortion	7
			Discordance and possible distortion	3
	Reject relationship (1)	Try to be considerate (1)	Discordance and adaptation	3

V. Low to very high affection, sexual "tries," "attempts," or "snuggles"	Don't want to be bothered (1)	Won't let me (1)	Discordance	3
	No sex perfectly OK (1)	We get along (1)	Concordance	3
	Like to snuggle (1)	Give in if she is tired (1)	Concordance	3
VI. Low to high affection and regular sexual intimacy	No problems (2)	No problems (2F)	Concordance	7
	Frustrated with mate's lack of affection (1)	Not as I should; can't talk about it (1F)	Discordance	3
	Bothered by mate's childlike affection (1)	I might be the weak one; distorts frequency (1)	Discordance and distortion	3
VII. High affection and sexual intimacy of 10 or more times per month	Sex OK but miss gifts he used to give (1)	Love it (1)	Adaptation and concordance	3
	Some resentment; feelings of being exploited; trying to accommodate mate (3)	No problem; enjoy it (2)	Discordance and distortion (adaptation and possible disorder)	7
		Try not to bother her and distorts frequency (1)	Discordance/adaptation and distortion	3

SOURCE: From "The Impact of Alzheimer's Disease on the Marital Relationship" by L. K. Wright, 1991, *The Gerontologist*, 31(2), p. 234. Copyright © The Gerontological Society of America. Reprinted with permission.
NOTE: F = Female spouse. Percentages do not add up to 100 due to rounding errors.

TABLE 5.4 Affection, Sexual Intimacy, Coping Themes, and Developmental Outcomes for Well Group Couples (*n* = 17)

Category/Relationship characterization	Coping Themes Female spouse (n)	Male spouse (n)	Developmental Outcomes Female spouse-Male spouse	% couples
I. No or rare affection, no sexual interest	Sex declines with age; spiritual and emotional more important (1)	Same (1)	Concordance	6
II. Moderate to high affection, no sexual interest	—	—		
III. No or rare affection, verbal expression of sexual interest	—	—		
IV. Low affection and verbal expression of sexual interest	Pain, refusal of intimacy; some doubt (1)	Still physically able; some regret (1)	Discordance	6
V. Moderate to high affection; some "tries" or very infrequent sexual intimacy	Sex declines with age; mutually affectionate (3)	Age; mutual affection; prostrate problem (2)	Concordance/adaptation	12
		She probably more affectionate (1)	Concordance/adaptation	6

VI. Low to high affection and regular sexual intimacy	Sex declines with age (4)	Declines with age (3)	Concordance/adaptation	18
	Frequency OK (6)	Physical problem (1)	Concordance/adaptation	6
	Frequency OK (2)	Frequency OK (6)	Concordance	35
		Medication side effects upsetting (1)		
		Frequency too low (1)	Adaptation	6
	Bantering over affection (same couples):			
	Mutually affectionate (9)	Mutual affection (8)	Adaptation and discordance	6
	I'm more affectionate (3)	I'm more affectionate (4)		
VII. High affection and sexual intimacy > 10 times per month	—	—		

one of only four others who considered the possibility of another relationship in case she became widowed. All other caregiver spouses (80%) and all of the afflicted spouses (100%) stated that they would never build a close relationship with another person. Category III, therefore, the combination of no or low affection, absence of actual intimacy but retained sexual interest, may be the most problematic in terms of coping and outcomes.

Category IV is similar to Category III except that affection is not absent or very low, but rather moderate or high; there is absence of actual intimacy, but continued interest in sexuality is expressed verbally. The coping themes in Category IV are either abstaining from sexual intimacy so as not to exploit the afflicted spouse or minimizing absence of sexual relations as "just one part of life." Only one caregiver in this category outright rejected a relationship with her husband, and he was very much aware of her feelings. However, similar to Category III, three afflicted spouses distorted the situation. The wife caregivers reported absence of sexual intimacy, while the respective afflicted husbands claimed to be sexually active ranging from "when she feels like it," to "once a month" to "every 2 weeks."

Category V relationships are characterized by low to very high affection and sexual gestures like "attempts" or "snuggles." For two caregiver spouses this situation was quite acceptable; only one stated that she did not want to be bothered. In all of the situations, the afflicted spouses were aware of the caregivers' feelings and gave congruent answers.

Category VI relationships are characterized by varying degrees of affection and regular sexual intimacy. This category includes the highest proportion of female afflicted spouses, possibly indicating that it is easier for male caregivers to retain a sexual relationship with a memory-impaired spouse. This is a very cautious interpretation, however, given the small number of female afflicted spouses in this study.

Two couples, each with a female afflicted spouse, reported no problems in their relationships, but one male caregiver complained about his wife's lack of affection; she was aware of her behavior but felt that she could not talk about it. Also in Category VI was a female caregiver who complained about her husband's child-like affection. It seems that he was not aware of his behavior, claiming initially higher sexual activity than his wife had reported (about 12 per month versus her report of 8 per month), but later he corrected himself and said "maybe twice a month."

Category VII, high affection and sexual intimacy of 10 or more times per month, is represented by male afflicted-female caregiver couples only. For one caregiver wife, this situation was acceptable; the couple had been highly sexually active in the past. However, the other caregivers voiced feelings of resentment and exploitation, particularly when, as in two cases, the afflicted husband seemed unaware of their feelings, claiming there were no problems and that they enjoyed it. In another case, however, the afflicted husband showed some awareness; he tried "not to bother her," and yet he claimed sexual activity of 12 to 14 times per month, while his caregiver wife reported 10.

Caregivers in Category VII also had the practical problem of finding suitable respite care. Most respite workers are female, and caregiver wives were reluctant to leave a sexually preoccupied mate alone at home with another female.

Well Group

When evaluating relationship patterns for well group couples (Table 5.4), rare or no affection, together with no sexual interest (Category I), can be agreeable to both spouses; age and concomitant physical changes were given as reasons. Relationship characterizations pertaining to Categories II and III identified for AD group couples were absent among well group couples.

Low affection and some retained interest in sexual matters (Category IV) resulted in doubt and some regrets for well group couples. This category perhaps shares some resemblance to Category III of the AD group because greater sexual interest is retained in one spouse than in the other. In the Alzheimer's situation, however, affection was not low but practically absent. Contrary to caregiver spouses, the well husband who voiced regrets was not seeking another intimate relationship (in fact, none of the well group couples did), but he engaged in many outside social activities separate from his wife's activities.

Categories V and VI are characterized by varying levels of affection and either very infrequent or regular sexual intimacy. Partners attributed decline in sexual activity to increasing age, and they adapted to limitations attributed to the husband's prostate problems. One male spouse in Category VI complained about medication side effects (on sexual performance), but his wife had adapted. Only one husband in Category VI said that his sexual appetite was stronger than his wife's. Overall, the couples were very much in tune with each other's wants and needs. Bantering over who was more affectionate was a friendly exchange and did not seem to indicate problems or conflicts. Category VII did not apply to well group couples.

HUMAN DEVELOPMENT RELATED
TO AFFECTION AND SEXUALITY

At any time during a married couple's life, biological, psychological, and sociocultural factors can impact on the affectional/sexual relationship, but even more so with advancing age. Thus a couple's intimate relationship is a reflection of human development. In this study, most well couples' relationships are characterized by low to high affection and regular sexual intimacy. Consistent with findings by other researchers, increasing age and physical limitations tended to decrease sexual activity, but, developmentally, there was high concordance and adaptation to any problems concerning intimacy. As shown in Table 5.4, this was the pattern for 88% of the couples; only 12% voiced some discordance.

In the presence of Alzheimer's disease, however, no dominant pattern can describe developmental outcomes. Only 42% of the relationships evidenced concordance and adaptation. Yet it is perhaps remarkable that even this many couples were similar to the well group. Absence of affection and sexual intimacy, just as for well spouses, was congruent with several of the AD couples' development, as indicated by their reference to the aging process.

Discordant relationships were related predominantly to either absence of sexual relations with retained sexual interest in the caregiver spouse and distortions by afflicted spouses or high sexual activity demanded by afflicted male spouses. Adaptation and control were difficult for the caregivers in the latter situations. Barusch (1988) reported that when it comes to sexual problems, caregiver spouses are unable to cope. What was meant by "sexual problems" was not defined. Quayhagen and Quayhagen (1988) were more specific; they reported that inappropriate sexual exposure by afflicted spouses is more stressful to caregiver wives than to caregiver husbands. Because in this study only couples with a male afflicted spouse had a pattern of high sexual activity (10 or more times per month), Quayhagen and Quayhagen's report may need to be reinterpreted. Perhaps more than sexual exposure is involved; perhaps at the same time, afflicted husbands make demands for sexual intimacy.

Very little information about this subject can be found in other research reports. In only one case report in the literature has an afflicted wife been described as exhibiting hypersexuality (Litz, Zeiss, & Davies, 1990). However, whether hypersexuality occurs less frequently or at similar rates in female versus male afflicted spouses is an unanswered question. Most caregiver studies simply do not report this information. It is also not known what causes high sexual activity. Monga, Monga, Raina, and Hardjasudarma (1986) reported hypersexuality in patients with poststroke seizure activity in right or left temporal lobes; this activity may indicate that hypersexuality is organically activated behavior. However, it is not known whether similar brain changes are involved for the small number of Alzheimer's disease afflicted persons.

It is also not known why, in this study, some afflicted spouses overreported frequency of sexual contacts or claimed to be sexually active when apparently they were not. Were they trying to convey some needs that they could not express in different words? Did their distortions represent wishful thinking based on a longing for closeness with the caregiver spouse? Or did these afflicted spouses try to deny problems and avoid embarrassment?

It is also possible that their distortions were the result of impaired cognition itself. We simply do not know.

And yet it is important to note that many afflicted spouses were quite aware of the feelings surrounding their intimate relationships. Even when they were rejected, they described their mates' feelings accurately and also expressed anger. In fact, 37% of all afflicted spouses were able "to take the attitude of the other" concerning affectional and sexual interactions with their spouses.

ASSESSMENT STRATEGIES AND INTERVENTION GUIDELINES

Assessment Strategies

Assessment of affection and sexuality needs to focus on three issues: (a) frequency of affectional and sexual expression between spouses, (b) agreement over affection and sexuality, and (c) problems concerning affection and sexuality. Assessment of affection and sexuality requires great sensitivity on the part of the health professional. Obviously the topic should not be introduced at the beginning of the assessment; some rapport needs to be established first. The topic may be introduced by acknowledging that affection and sexuality are very personal issues and that spouses may refuse to answer any question. When spouses have a problem, they will be glad that someone is addressing this issue. Refusal to answer questions probably will be rare. In this study, only one male from the well group did not want to answer one of the open-ended questions.

It is highly recommended that spouses be interviewed separately for questions pertaining to affection and sexuality. This not only prevents embarrassment but also provides the interviewer with an assessment of how congruent or divergent spouses are in their own assessment of the relationship.

To assess frequency of affection, the revised affection subscale of the Dyadic Adjustment Rating Scale (Spanier & Thompson, 1982;

Wright, 1991a) will be useful. (Scale items and scoring methods are described at the beginning of this chapter.) The scale items will help focus the interview for additional open-ended questions. Past and present problems will emerge, including agreement over affection, and this knowledge will be important for planning interventions.

The topic of sexuality may be introduced by stating that, in general, sexual activity tends to decline as people age but that there are great individual differences. Then the most direct question is "How often per month do you and your spouse have sexual relations?" This question, as well as the subsequent question "How much do you and your spouse agree on sexual issues?" will bring out present and past problems.

To assess clinical problems, additional questions need to focus on type of medications taken, absence or presence of dyspareunia (painful intercourse), and cystitis (bladder and urine infections). Particular attention needs to be paid to hypertensive (high blood pressure) medications because they are known to cause erection problems in males. However, a diet poor in iron and excess use of alcohol and smoking also can cause this problem. Absence of hormone replacement therapy is a likely cause of dyspareunia in female spouses, and poor hygiene, together with frequent sexual intercourse, may be the cause of recurrent bladder infections.

Intervention Guidelines

Relatively healthy spouses rarely will need interventions for issues pertaining to affectional expression. These couples seem to work things out just fine. A common sense book such as *Sexual Health in Later Life* (Walz & Blum, 1987) may be recommended to provide additional knowledge. If sexual problems seem related to medical problems and particularly to medication side effects, a check-up with a physician needs to be advised.

Intervening with problems experienced by afflicted spouse-caregiver spouse dyads is much more difficult. No doubt the quality of couples' past marital relationships will affect caregivers' present feelings (Robinson, 1989, 1990a). Hugging, kissing, embracing, and other affectional gestures seem to have a calming effect on afflicted spouses (Wright, 1991a). But if caregivers are emotionally unable to engage in this type of behavior, then they need to be supported in their decision. An intervention strategy of involving other family members in expressing affection to the afflicted person may be tried, but this may not be successful. When an afflicted spouse has excessive sexual desires, even the most loving spouse will need help. Four intervention strategies may be considered in such situations: (a) If the caregiver spouse is emotionally able and willing, relieving the afflicted spouse manually may be suggested, (b) referral to a physician for possible medication control may be arranged, (c) general hygiene and techniques for reducing trauma to the female urethra may be taught, and (d) arrangements for a male respite worker may be made by working with agency personnel. To elaborate on the third point, the techniques for preventing or minimizing problems are (a) washing both spouses' genital areas before and after intercourse, (b) using a water soluble lubricant (e. g., K-Y lubricating jelly, not Vaseline), (c) letting the female spouse assume the "on top" position during intercourse to reduce trauma to the urethra, and (d) drinking a large glassful of water after intercourse and at the first sign of bladder irritations.

But caregiver spouses also have needs, and most of these go unmet. Their needs have to be acknowledged. Support group leaders should consider seriously the creation of separate spouse-only caregiver groups where issues of affection and sexuality can be more openly discussed than in groups also attended by caregivers who are adult children or even grandchildren. Solutions to all problems may not be found, but to ask about them, instead of pretending the subject does not exist, is the beginning of an intervention.

Commitment and the Marital Relationship

INTRODUCTION

The words *commitment and marriage* evoke images of a couple pledging traditional wedding vows: "For better, for worse, in sickness and in health, until death do us part." Faithfulness is inherent in this pledge. For older couples, gratitude is added to the pledge because of shared memories for good times in the past. Simmel (1950) distinguished between faithfulness and gratitude and eloquently clarified their meaning. *Faithfulness,* Simmel stated, is enduring love, and it might be called "the inertia of the soul. It keeps the soul on the path on which it started, even after the original occasion that led it onto it no longer exists" (Simmel, 1950, p. 380). *Gratitude,* however, is not the actual return of a gift, but it places the receiver's consciousness "into a certain permanent position with respect to the giver, and makes him dimly envisage the inner infinity of a relations" (Simmel, 1950, p. 392). Gratitude, in other words, is irredeemable: One stays obliged to someone who has earned our thanks. Gratitude, Simmel stated, "is the moral memory of mankind, and without faithfulness, "society simply could not exist" (Simmel, 1950, p. 379).

Most couples in this study expressed sentiments of faithfulness and gratitude or commitment to their marriage. Even couples for whom it was a second marriage (6 years duration in one case, 12 years in another) expressed sentiments of commitment. It undoubtedly is an important issue, but trying to measure such sentiments is more difficult. The couples' shared past, from the time they met and married, and their present feelings about each other and the future have to be taken into consideration.

EXPLORING COMMITMENT
TO THE MARITAL RELATIONSHIP

In light of the importance of couples' shared past when trying to measure present and future commitment to the relationship, three major questions were posed in an effort to incorporate the time element: (a) Has there been a change in commitment to the spouse as a uniquely valued person over the course of the couples' marriage? (b) How do both groups of couples rate commitment to the future of their relationship? and (c) Are past marital happiness, valuing the spouse as a unique person in the present, and feelings about the future related?

Has There Been a Change in Commitment
to the Spouse as a Uniquely Valued Person
Over the Course of the Couples' Marriage?

To assess whether change in commitment to the spouse as a uniquely valued person had occurred over the course of a couple's marriage, two questions were posed to each spouse (at different times in the interview sequence): (a) Why did you marry your spouse? and (b) Why have you stayed married to your spouse?

These two questions are based on the work by Swensen and Trahaug (1985), who found significantly fewer marital problems in long-term marriages when the partners' commitment is based on valuing the spouse as a unique person versus valuing marriage as an institution. For example, the answer "It's natural to

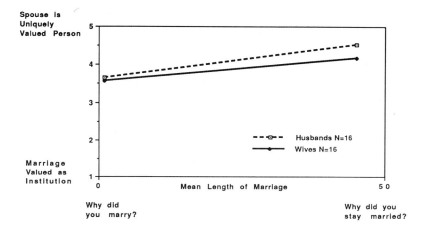

Figure 6.1. Commitment Over Time: Well Couples

get (stay) married" would indicate a spouse's commitment to marriage as an institution, while the answer "There was (is) no one like him (or her)" would indicate that the spouse is perceived as a uniquely valued person.

The spouses' answers were rated on a continuum of 1 through 5, with 4 and 5 indicating that the spouse was valued as a unique person, 1 and 2 that marriage was valued as an institution; 3 was given to answers that were equally strong in both sentiments, for example, "I love him. We made a lifetime commitment." Four independent raters assigned the numerical values to the spouses' answers; agreement among the raters was high. Figure 6.1 summarizes well group spouses' answers. Figure 6.2 presents those given by spouses in the AD group.

The first question, "Why did you marry?" is considered to be the beginning of a couple's relationship and is shown on the left side of the horizontal line (the *x* axis) of each graph. The second question, "Why have you stayed married?" is considered to be the present and anchors the right side of the line. Thus the horizontal axis represents a time interval; it is the couples' mean length of marriage, which was 45 years for the well group. As

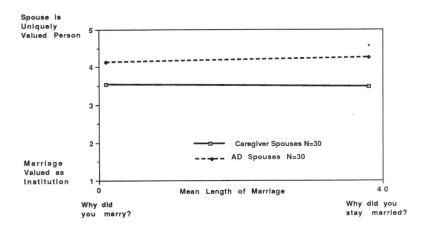

Figure 6.2. Commitment Over Time: AD Couples

can be noted in Figure 6.1, husbands and wives from the well group gave very similar answers for Time 1, the beginning of their relationship (3.6 for wives, 3.7 for husbands). At Time 2, the present, husbands were slightly higher in their commitment to the spouse as a uniquely valued person, but the difference between husbands (4.5) and wives (4.2) is not significant. However, a significant change did occur over the course of their marriage: Well group spouses increased significantly in the direction of valuing the spouse as a unique person.

In Figure 6.2, the graph for the AD group, a different picture emerges. Here the time interval for the couples' mean length of marriage represents 38 years. For Time 1, afflicted spouses' answers indicate high commitment to the spouse as a person (4.1), while answers by caregiver spouses (3.5) are similar to those given by well group couples. For Time 2, the present, afflicted spouses again indicate higher commitment to the spouse as a unique person than do caregivers (4.3 versus 3.5, respectively), and this difference between spouses is statistically significant. However, no significant change occurred over time for either spouse in the AD group even though well group spouses had changed significantly. Yet the remarkable finding is that even though caregiver spouses did not increase in commitment, they stayed at the same level of commitment. They valued the mate as a unique person despite cognitive impairment and sometimes difficult behaviors in the afflicted spouse. One might have expected that their commitment would have moved more in the direction of valuing marriage as an institution, the marriage vows and faithfulness that Simmel (1950) described. Indeed many caregivers did mention their wedding vows "for better or worse, in sickness and in health," but they also added, "I still love him (or her)." They were, in other words, hanging on to an image of the spouse as a unique person.

How Do Both Groups of Couples Rate Commitment to the Future of Their Relationship?

Commitment to the future of the relationship was assessed with a 6 point measure that is part of Spanier and Thompson's (1982) Dyadic Adjustment Rating Scale. Spouses were asked to rate feelings about the future of their relationship, with response options ranging from *I will go to any length to see that the relationship succeeds* (6) to *There is no more that I can do to keep the relationship going* (1). A summary of these ratings is presented in Table 6.1

Husbands and wives from the well group gave very similar answers, and both were high in their commitment to the future of the relationship. Couples from the AD group, however, differed. Caregivers were significantly lower in their commitment than afflicted spouses, and they also were significantly lower in commitment to the future of the relationship than well group spouses. Lower in commitment to the future but stable in commitment to the spouse as a unique person—is this a contradiction? Perhaps not, as will be shown in the next section.

TABLE 6.1 Commitment to the Future of the Relationship by Group and Couple Comparison

Group comparison (means)	
Alzheimer's group	Well group
n = 30	n = 17
4.7*	5.5

		Couple comparison (means)	
Caregivers	Afflicted	Female	Male
n = 30	n = 30	n = 17	n = 17
4.7**	5.6	5.4	5.3

NOTE: Possible range of scores: 6 = highest commitment, 1 = lowest commitment.
*p = < .05; **p = .01.

Are Past Marital Happiness, Valuing the Spouse as a Unique Person, and Feelings About the Future Related?

Past marital happiness was assessed by asking spouses to rate the degree of past happiness, "all things considered." This measure was adapted from Spanier and Thompson's (1982) Dyadic Adjustment Rating Scale. Response options ranged from *perfect* (7) to *extremely unhappy* (1). Spouses were told that the middle point, *happy* (4), represents the amount of happiness in most relationships.

Interestingly, no significant differences between ratings of past marital happiness were found when comparing caregivers, afflicted spouses, and well group husbands and wives. Most spouses rated their past marital relationship as *very happy* (5), a few gave it a low *fairly unhappy* (2) rating, and some indicated it as *perfect* (7). The average for all spouses was 4.9. This finding is important because it helps support the supposition that comparisons between the two groups of couples made throughout this book are valid; the couples seem to have been similar before Alzheimer's disease changed the relationship of caregiver and afflicted spouses.

To answer whether past marital happiness is related to valuing the spouse as a unique person in the present and to feelings about the future of the relationship, correlation analyses were

TABLE 6.2 Correlations Between Past Marital Happiness, Valuing the Spouse as a Unique Person, Commitment to the Future of the Relationship, Impairment Levels of Afflicted Spouses, and Caregiver Health (n = 30 Caregivers).

	(1)	(2)	(3)	(4)	(5)	(6)	(7)	(8)
Caregiver's past marital happiness (1)	1							
Caregiver's view of spouse as unique person (2)	.539**	1						
Caregivers' commitment to future of relationship (3)	.225	.189	1					
AD spouse's Mini-Mental (4)	.191	.084	−.098	1				
AD spouse's GDS (5)	−.185	−.137	.261	−.899**	1			
AD spouse's length of illness (6)	−.17	−.29	.177	−.453**	.58***	1		
Caregiver's physical health (7)	−.061	.21	.387*	−.101	.167	.004	1	
Caregiver's depressed moods (8)	−.282	−.161	−.381*	−.096	.019	−.01	−.581***	1

NOTE: *p < .05; **p < .01; ***p < .001.

performed for the variables in question. No relationships were found between any of the variables for husbands and wives from the well group or for the afflicted spouses.

But the most important question is whether past marital happiness influences commitment in caregiver spouses. Indeed, as shown in Table 6.2, those caregivers who had high past marital happiness were high in valuing the spouse as a unique person in the present (r = .539, p < .01). These were the caregivers who—even in the presence of Alzheimer's disease—were hanging on to an image of the past. Yet past marital happiness did not influence their feelings about the future, nor did valuing the spouse as a unique person now, in the present, influence feelings about the future.

Commitment to the future of the relationship is an important issue when considering that all of the caregivers in this study still lived together with the afflicted spouse and provided care at home. In the future, however, an afflicted spouse could be placed into a nursing home. The finding that neither past marital happiness nor present feelings for the spouse as a unique person influenced the caregivers' commitment to the future is, therefore, somewhat disturbing. The most obvious question that comes to mind is: Has the afflicted spouse's severity of illness a more important impact on feelings about the future than past marital happiness or still loving the spouse as a unique person? This hypothesis was not supported when afflicted spouses' memory and functional impairment (Mini-Mental State and Reisberg's Global Deterioration Scale) and length of illness were evaluated in relation to the caregivers' commitment to the future. However, two other important variables were considered: the caregivers' own physical health and depressed moods. It was found that the better the caregivers' self-rated physical health and the more positive their moods, the higher their commitment to the future of the relationship ($r = .387$ and $r = .381$, $p < .05$; see Table 6.2). Here, then, are important clues that have implications for planning immediate interventions and anticipating future needs. Why? Because commitment to the future requires energy. If the caregiver's own physical and emotional health is failing, then despite past marital happiness, despite still valuing the spouse as a unique person, and despite faithfulness and gratitude, to use Simmel's (1950) words, commitment to the future of the relationship is affected.

HUMAN DEVELOPMENT AND COMMITMENT TO MARRIAGE

Commitment is the essence of long-term relationships; it captures the time element in human development. Commitment can be mutually satisfying and beneficial to partners and can sustain the relationship in times of crisis. Well group couples in this study epitomize mutually satisfying commitment and the "best as yet to be": With the passing of time, husbands and wives increasingly value each other as unique persons, and they have high commitment to the future of their relationship.

Afflicted spouses also have high commitment to the future and high appraisal of the spouse as a unique person, but their feelings do not match those reported by caregivers. Afflicted spouses are quite aware that the spouse is the most important person in their lives. As one put it, "After all, she is very important around here." It seems that in everything afflicted spouses express, they communicate their high need for closeness or attachment.

For caregivers, faithfulness and gratitude are remarkably powerful sentiments in maintaining the image of the spouse as a valued person. However, another life dimension exerts its influence: The caregiver's own health creates asynchronies between psychological commitment and physical limitations. Caregivers cannot expect help from the other spouse. This realistic assessment of the future, influenced by knowledge about their own health, is particularly poignant when noting that other studies have documented repeatedly that spouse caregivers, even if old and frail themselves, "are the last to relinquish care [of a mate] to professionals" (Colerick & George, 1986, p. 496). When a caregiver spouse says, "There is no more I can do," we need to pay attention.

ASSESSMENT STRATEGIES AND INTERVENTION GUIDELINES

Assessment Strategies

Health professionals interested in assessing the quality of a couple's relationship may focus on three issues: (a) commitment to the spouse as a unique person, (b) past marital happiness, and (c) commitment to the future of the relationship. Commitment to the spouse can be assessed with two questions: "Why did you marry?" and "Why have you stayed married?" These two questions help anchor past and present (Swensen & Trahaug, 1985). One of these questions should be asked early in the interview sequence, the other one later, and answers should be recorded verbatim. Experience has shown that it is fairly easy to rate the expressed sentiments on a 5-point continuum of *marriage valued as an institution* versus *the spouse valued as a unique person*. It is particularly important to make this assessment if caregivers give an indication of having "given up" on the spouse, as discussed in Chapter 3.

Past marital happiness can be assessed with a 7-point, easy-to-respond-to measure (Spanier & Thompson, 1982) described earlier in this chapter. If a low score is obtained, additional questions about past problems may be raised. But how far back is the past? To obtain an approximate equal time frame for couples in this study, the AD group was asked to think about the time prior to the onset of illness, and the well group was asked to think about the time prior to one or both spouses' retirement. The reference point for both groups thus represented a time when spouses did not experience a constant togetherness, and the mean number of years they used as point of reference was, in fact, about the same.

Commitment to the future of the relationship can be assessed by asking "How do you feel about the future of your relationship with your spouse?" Six response options can be listed, and the spouse can be asked to choose one: *I will go to any length to see that our relationship succeeds* (6), *I will do all I can to see that it does* (5), *I will do my fair share to see that it does* (4), *I can't do much more than I am doing now to keep the relationship going* (3), *I refuse to do any more than I am doing now to keep the relationship going* (2), and *There is no more that I can do to keep the relationship going* (1) (Spanier & Thompson, 1982). Commitment to the future is an important assessment question because spouses are realistic and honest when they project into the future. Indeed, in a follow-up study, low commitment to the future of the relationship at the initial interview was found to be a significant predictor for nursing home placement 2 years later (Wright, 1991b). However, along with assessing future commitment, an assessment of the caregivers' physical and emotional health needs to be made.

A number of tools for assessing health are available, ranging from a single question to more comprehensive measures. For example, self-rated health—"Please rate your own health as either excellent, good, fair, or poor"—has been found to be a valid and reliable indicator (Liang, 1986). If time permits or if indicated by this initial screening, additional assessments may be made. A more comprehensive physical health measure that was used in this study is the Multiple Assessment Inventory (MAI; Lawton, Moss, Fulcomer, & Kleban, 1982; Weinberger et al., 1986). Qualified health professionals will want to perform a direct physical assessment as needed. Frequently used and suitable depression measures are the Geriatric Depression Scale (Yesavage et al., 1983) and the Short Zung Interviewer Assisted Scale (Tucker, Ogle, Davinson, & Eilenberg, 1986, 1987).

Intervention Guidelines

We cannot change the past, and we can hardly influence feelings of faithfulness and gratitude. However, commitment to the future is related to the caregiver's own health, and health care professionals can intervene when the caregiver's physical and emotional health is threatened. The emotional impact of caregiving is well recognized, but the impact on physical health is less clear (Schulz, Visantainer, & Williamson, 1990). Caregivers may rate their health as poor, but they do not necessarily seek medical help (Snyder & Keefe, 1985).

As a general rule, therefore, anytime an afflicted spouse is evaluated in a clinic or during a home visit, the caregiver's health should be assessed, and interventions should be started if necessary. In addition, agency personnel who coordinate respite services and support group leaders who have regular contacts with caregivers can put literal meaning into the polite social exchange "Take care of yourself." Plans for seeking help for specific problems need to be discussed, and follow-up inquiries need to be made. If the caregiver's health can be maintained, there is a good chance that the afflicted spouse will remain at home. Unfortunately the health of some caregivers will decline to the point where caring for an afflicted spouse at home becomes unrealistic. In such situations, nursing home placement has to be considered (unless another family member can take over the responsibilities of caregiving).

When a caregiver is faced with the decision to institutionalize an afflicted spouse, all available information and assistance must be provided. Key issues to be considered are (a) financial arrangements, (b) type of nursing home, and (c) support to the caregiver during and after the decision phase.

As already stressed in Chapter 2, financial arrangements require expert advice. The 1990 Office of Technology (OTA) report "Confused Minds, Burdened Families" concluded that because long-term care has many sources of funding with complex and changing rules that differ from state to state, it is very difficult for caregivers to obtain accurate information. It is therefore beyond the scope of this book to give precise guidelines, but some of the most important points will be addressed.

First, if a private insurance policy exists, it should be evaluated by an expert, preferably by a social worker or geriatric nurse practitioner. Some policies do cover long-term nursing home or "custodial" care; others have a number of exclusion criteria.

When private insurance for long-term care is not present, the question whether Medicare or Medicaid will pay for nursing home care arises. The answer is not a simple yes or no. Some basic explanations and distinctions need to be made.

Any person aged 65 or older who is entitled to Social Security benefits (a person with a work history and who has paid sufficient Social Security taxes) is entitled to the federal health insurance program Medicare, Part A and Part B. Part A is the hospital insurance (which has several "deductible" regulations depending on length of hospital stay). Part B is the Supplemental Medical insurance that people may opt to drop (but most people do not). Part B pays for a large portion of physician and outpatient services (80% of the approved amount after $100 deductible) (Special Committee on Aging, 1990).

Medicare Part A will pay for care in a *skilled* nursing home for a limited number of days if a memory-impaired person has, *in addition*, a physical condition that requires treatment *and* that has potential for cure. The rules for payment are as follows: A prior hospital stay of 3 days or entry within 30 days after a hospital discharge are required (Mitchell, 1991). For the first 20 days, 100% of the skilled nursing home stay costs are covered. From the 21st to the 100th day, all but $81.50 a day are covered. This deductible amount *may* be paid by Medicaid to persons eligible for both Medicare and Medicaid. However, Medicare will not pay for nursing home care if the person is "only" demented. This is where Medicaid plays a role.

Medicaid is a state-federal program for people who cannot pay for health care costs. By law, the Health Care Financing Administration (HCFA) pays approximately 55% of the states' health care, and individual states and counties pay the rest. Medicaid will pay for nursing home care, but many rules govern a couple's available assets.

To determine eligibility for Medicaid payments, a caseworker at the local Department of Social Services (DSS) will take a "snapshot" of the couple's assets, determine how assets are to be divided, and evaluate each spouse's monthly income.

The caregiver spouse, from now on referred to as the "at-home" spouse, gets to keep the house and one vehicle. All other assets are then counted. As of July 1, 1992, the at-home spouse may keep all assets if they do not exceed $13,926. If the assets are over this amount, they are split between the at-home and the institutionalized spouse. For example, if total assets are $100,000, each spouse gets $50,000. If the couple's assets are much higher, then the maximum amount the at-home spouse may keep is $66,480. The institutionalized spouse's portion of the assets is used to pay for nursing home care expenses before Medicaid will pay (this is referred to as "spending down" assets in order to become eligible).

Monthly income in the form of pensions or from other sources also is considered. A pension solely in the name of the at-home spouse cannot be considered for nursing home payment of the other spouse. If the pension is in the institutionalized spouse's name, he or she gets to keep $30 per month; the rest goes toward nursing home payments. However, if the income of the at-home spouse is less than $1,149 per month, then DSS may deem up to that amount to the spouse at home from the pension of the institutionalized spouse. If the at-home spouse's expenses for mortgage or rent, food, and so forth exceed $1,149, then DSS may deem up to $1,600 per month to the at home spouse. In such cases, however, some restrictions on what Medicaid will cover for the institutionalized spouse come into effect.

As can be seen, even these very basic current regulations have many "*if*'s." Every situation is slightly different, and laws change. The most important intervention for a caregiver spouse in the transition phase of in-home to nursing home care is to make a referral to a professional who specializes in eligibility criteria. Geriatric nurse practitioners or clinical nurse specialists, social workers, and caseworkers at the Department of Social Services are some of the most informed people in this area.

The next important issue is the selection of a nursing home. This decision requires knowledge about such factors as staffing patterns, type of program offered, and nursing home licensing rules. An excellent selection guide that can be used by caregivers has been described by Gwyther (1988), and the complex issue of choosing a nursing home is extensively discussed in Chapter 5 of OTA's (1990) report "Confused Minds, Burdened Families."

Finally the caregiver spouse needs emotional support during the decision-making phase but probably even more so after the afflicted spouse has been institutionalized (Rosenthal & Dawson, 1991). Professionals previously involved with the couple may drop out of the picture, and the nursing home staff now become central. The latter will need to be sensitive to the continuing bond between couples. A plan of care that involves previous caregivers and that makes use of their accumulated knowledge about the "patient" has to be designed. Maas, Buckwalter, and Kelley (1991a, 1991b), on the basis of findings with special units for Alzheimer's disease patients, have stressed the importance of involving close family members in the planning of care, as well as allowing them to participate in the actual care if they wish.

SEVEN

Conclusions

In the foregoing chapters, several dimensions of the marital relationship were explored. They included household responsibilities, tension, companionship, affection and sexuality, and commitment. In this chapter, key findings will be summarized, coping strategies as measured with the Jalowiec Coping Scale (Jalowiec, 1988) will be presented, conclusions about human development for both groups of couples will be attempted, and finally the most important implications for practice derived from this study will be stated.

SUMMARY OF FINDINGS

The general character of the marital relationship is profoundly different for the two groups. Shared responsibilities, low tension, enjoyment of each other's companionship, and high affectional and regular sexual expression characterize well group couples. The capacity to "take the attitude of the other" is the hallmark of their relationship, and with the passing of time, spouses increasingly value each other as unique persons. The overall developmental outcome for well couples is a concordant relationship.

In the presence of Alzheimer's disease, however, characteristics of the marital relationship are not identical for partners. Caregiver spouses carry major household responsibilities alone, they often use tension control and displacement as a means of dealing with emotional strains, they have a need for substitute companionship, and they either accept or are frustrated over the lost sexual relationship or are resentful of excessive sexual demands. Most caregivers retain the capacity to take the attitude of the afflicted spouse, and this contributes to their commitment to stay in the relationship. Caregivers do not change in the direction of commitment to marriage as an institution; rather they hang on to an image of the spouse as a valued person.

Afflicted spouses view household responsibilities as unproblematic, they perceive low tension, and they have a high need for a close, clinging type of companionship. Expression of affection may be low or anxiously high, while sexual expression tends to be lost but in a few cases becomes exaggerated. Afflicted spouses show varying degrees of capacity to take the attitude of the other, and when they do, it influences their actions: They withdraw from the relationship when they sense rejection, and they restrict other social contacts when interactions are perceived as too complex. They recognize that their spouse is the most important person in their life, and their commitment is based on high dependency needs.

The overall developmental outcome for couples in the Alzheimer's group cannot be described with a single adjective. Rather it is a committed-dependent relationship that spans outcomes of adaptation and control, as well as distortion and disorder.

COPING STRATEGIES
BASED ON THE JALOWIEC COPING SCALE

Throughout this book, developmental outcomes of adaptation or distortion, control or disorder, concordance or discordance were identified for specific dimensions of the marital relationship. These outcomes do not simply happen; rather they result from behavioral, cognitive, and emotional efforts of individuals confronted with trying to solve difficult life situations. In other words, outcomes are influenced by coping and by all the social interactions inherent in coping. How spouses in this study coped with specific marital issues has been described. The descriptions were based on their own reports, their own words, or the qualitative approach of documenting coping.

Another method of documenting coping is the quantitative approach, which attempts to measure, with a standardized scale, how often people make cognitive, behavioral, and emotional efforts "to master, tolerate or reduce external and internal demands and conflicts between them" (Folkman & Lazarus, 1980, p. 223; Pearlin & Schooler, 1978).

Several conceptual perspectives of coping exist; these include coping as personality traits, coping as ego defense mechanisms, and coping as demands to specific situations (Antonovsky, 1987; Haan, 1977; Lazarus, Averill, & Opton, 1974; Lieberman & Tobin, 1983; McCubbin, Cauble, & Patterson, 1982; Menninger, 1963; Moos, 1977; Pearlin, Mullan, Semple, & Skaff, 1990; Ray, Lindop, & Gibson, 1982). The last, coping as demands to specific situations, was considered to be an appropriate perspective because an afflicted spouse's illness requires situation-specific coping.

The Jalowiec Coping Scale (Jalowiec, 1988), which was used in this study, is congruent with this perspective. The scale has three subconcepts: confrontive, emotive, and palliative coping. These three types of coping strategies represent behavioral, emotional, and cognitive efforts made by people in response to specific situational demands. Spouses were asked to relate coping strategies listed on the scale to their marital relationship. Response options for each coping item ranged from doing it *almost always* (5) to *never* (1).

Caregiver spouses and well group couples completed the coping scale as a paper-and-pencil test. Afflicted spouses were given assistance with completing the scale. The interviewer read each scale item aloud and pointed to response options. The forms had large, bold print so that afflicted spouses could easily reread or repeat the items and point to answers. Following completion of the scale, spouses were asked to comment on a number of specific items—for example, "When you checked that you always 'actively change the situation,' what specifically have you done to change the situation?" This line of questioning brought to light a conceptually important (although to the interviewer, initially very frustrating) issue: The Alzheimer's afflicted spouses kept saying, "That depends on the situation. I really don't have any (or many big) problems." And when they gave examples of what they had done to change the situation, they referred back to their past working lives.

The well group spouses also said repeatedly, "Well, that depends on the situation," and in fact commented that they may have contradicted themselves in answering the scale items. The specific examples they gave tended to focus on problems concerning broader family relationships—for example, on problems their grown children or grandchildren currently were experiencing, or on conflicts among volunteer workers with whom they associated, or on past or present work experiences if still employed. They rarely considered their marital relationship as requiring attention with specific coping responses. Marital conflict was so low that talking things out or letting things be were adequate ways of dealing with problems.

It was only the caregiver spouses who focused on the marital relationship, and they related specific coping strategies to the presence of illness. But even caregivers added occasionally, "When I answered that questions, I thought about my daughter."

This discovery required rethinking the measurement of coping with a standardized scale. It led to the realization that the interviews confirmed the theoretical perspective that had been argued to begin with: Coping *is* situation specific, and it is only when difficulties, crises (asynchronies) occur that people activate specific behavioral, cognitive, or emotional strategies (Pearlin & Schooler, 1978). Well group spouses did not have problematic marriages, and the world of Alzheimer's afflicted spouses was— perhaps as a way of coping—kept unproblematic.

Only for caregivers can findings based on the standardized scale be considered an indication of marital coping. More accurately, the findings represent a global characterization of coping responses used for dealing with multifaceted marriage problems. For well

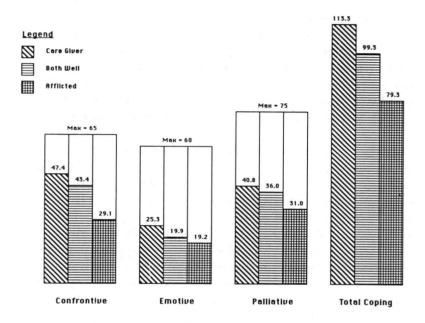

Figure 7.1. Comparison of Means Cores for Coping Strategies by Caregiver, Well, and Afflicted Spouses

group spouses the coping strategies reported possibly may represent certain personality traits (Antonovsky, 1987; Lazarus et al., 1974), although testing this assumption is beyond the scope of this study. For afflicted spouses, coping may represent defensive ego processes (Haan, 1977; Menninger, 1963; Ray et al., 1982), but their ego defenses are limited by impaired cognitive functioning.

With this important distinction as to the meaning of coping measured with a quantitated scale, a comparison of coping strategies as reported by caregiver, afflicted, and well spouses is presented in Figure 7.1. The graph shows the maximum possible score for each subscale of coping and the average (mean) score reported by caregivers, well group, and afflicted spouses.

Husbands and wives from the well group did not differ in their use of coping strategies, but they did differ from caregiver spouses. Caregiver spouses used significantly more coping strategies in total, and they used significantly more confrontive, emotive, and palliative coping. Caregivers seemed to use any means that could possibly help them in their situation.

By contrast, the lowest number of coping strategies was reported by afflicted spouses. Confrontive coping and palliative coping were their most common modes, yet, interestingly, afflicted spouses did not differ in emotive coping from well group spouses. This finding requires a closer look at the items measuring the subconcepts.

Emotive coping strategies included such items as getting nervous, worrying, taking tension out on others, expecting the worst, getting mad, wanting to be alone, and blaming others. Such behaviors require recognition of discomfort, precisely what the Alzheimer's afflicted person guards against perceiving. But in addition, these coping strategies have a negative connotation. Neither afflicted persons, nor caregivers, nor well group spouses readily admitted such thinking, feeling, or behavior: Emotive coping was the least used coping strategy reported by all.

Confrontive coping, the most frequently reported strategy for all groups, included such statements as seeking comfort or help from others, discussing the problem, seeking information, maintaining control, and engaging in activities. These were items that afflicted spouses seemed to understand in terms of their *past* work experience. Only repeated questioning would yield answers related to *now.*

Palliative coping included such items as not worrying, hoping for improvement, laughing it off, accepting the situation, praying, letting someone else solve the problem, doing nothing, and waiting it out. These were nonthreatening statements, and a number of the afflicted spouses agreed with the wording, saying, "That might be a good way of handling it." Others again said that they really did not have anything to worry about. The afflicted spouses' overall limitation in approaching or dealing with problems is demonstrated graphically with Figure 7.1.

Asynchronies remain unrecognized or unacknowledged, and thus coping becomes limited.

It also is shown in the graph that when the situation is defined as crisis or asynchrony, people will use more cognitive, emotional, and behavioral strategies than at any other time. It is the caregivers who experience the most asynchronized life dimensions, and energies seem to be released through this experience: Caregivers use more coping strategies than any other group. Whether certain coping strategies are better than others, "right or wrong" is not the issue; even crying and blaming may be appropriate responses to specific situations. This assertion is based on the fact that, overall, caregivers coped remarkably well.

HUMAN DEVELOPMENT AND PERSON-ENVIRONMENT INTERACTION

Throughout this book, findings related to specific aspects of the marital relationship have been interpreted within Riegel's (1979) dialectical theory of human development. Other theorists who built on Riegel's work have used different terminology. The words *life span developmental theory, contextualism,* and *epigenetic-probabilistic human development* can be found in the literature. Life span developmental theorists (Baltes, 1979; Brandtstaedter, 1984) emphasize successive change as persons age; but in contrast to theorists who describe life as a series of predetermined stages, life span developmentalists acknowledge the influence of person-environment interactions. Contextualism as a theory of human development (Lerner, 1985) gives greater emphasis to person-environment interactions and less to biological and aging influences. Contextualism and the epigenetic-probabilistic theory of human development (Lerner & Kauffman, 1985) have identical assumptions. *Epigenetic-probabilistic development* means that factors above and beyond genetics influence outcomes. Propositions of the epigenetic-probabilistic theory can be summarized as follows: Although human development involves successive and organized biological changes across the life span, dynamic interactions occur between person and environment.

Something new emerges from these interactions (the dialectic), and hence developmental outcomes are flexible and not predetermined (Lerner & Kauffman, 1985). Genetic and biological factors, in other words, interact with environmental factors, and great importance is ascribed to actions taken by individuals to influence their environment. These propositions are congruent with Riegel's (1979) earlier writings.

But can findings from this study support an epigenetic-probabilistic theory of human development? It seems that the influence of unusual biological factors has to be acknowledged. Namely the internal organization of an individual human being can become chaotic due to illness, and such an occurrence has profound implications for further human development for that individual. However, inner-biological or physical limitations that are not of chaotic proportions allow for person-environment interactions and development over time. The relatively healthy couples in this study integrated physical illness into their lives, adapted to them through environmental restructuring (e. g., moving to a different location, changing activities), or planned ahead for eventual widowhood in an organized manner that reflects life span development thinking.

For caregivers, a spouse's illness became a major environmental influence requiring major reorganizations of their lives. If one defines *development* as "a process of interactions which from the outside transforms the organism as he transforms the external conditions through his own activities" (Riegel, 1973, p. 5), then caregiver spouses were developing. They were transformed from the outside in, and they actively changed the external conditions of their environments. For example, they took charge of household responsibilities, they used many tension-reducing strategies, and they looked for, and at times used, support services. Their thoughts were focused predominantly on the present, although some projected into the future. Eventual widowhood was envisioned, and the realization that to some extent the process of aloneness had already begun. This realization of diminishing social contacts, together with an afflicted spouse's demanding or tiresome behaviors, created a need to escape and to be with other people. Consequently some caregiver spouses were beginning to enlarge their social environments, again demonstrating that they actively changed their external conditions in response to perceived asynchronies.

Overall, then, it can be stated with confidence that something new emerges from person-environment interactions and that human development is not predetermined. Furthermore people integrate experiences into their overall life plans in an organized manner—unless inner biological events are of catastrophic proportions as Riegel (1979) had already recognized.

The final issue to be addressed, therefore, is whether the term *development* still applies to persons who have Alzheimer's disease. As has been repeatedly noted, the afflicted spouses' definition of the situation is predominantly that of a nonproblematic world, and for each marital dimension assessed, only approximately one third of the afflicted spouses evidenced the capacity to take the attitude of the other spouse. Trying to explain this phenomenon within a dialectical, probabilistic theory of human development does not mean that pathological (brain structure) changes are dismissed as unimportant. The disease is recognized as causal influence on the afflicted person's functioning. To state it in the words of a caregiver wife, it is recognized that the "brain isn't working anymore." The explanation attempted here will focus on the interactional processes between such persons and their environment.

If, as Riegel has argued, life difficulties, crises, or asynchronies are major determinants of development, then, conversely, it can be argued that as the ability to perceive problems deteriorates, human development declines and eventually will stop. Such reasoning would get to the heart of a dialectical theory of human development, of person-environment interaction and resulting transformations versus a theory of development with predetermined stages toward a certain end condition (McCulloch, 1981).

But why should the ability to perceive asynchronies influence the capacity to develop? It can be argued that development requires energy and that afflicted persons lose energy input from the environment as their perceptions become more and more constricted. At first, the loss occurs cognitively in terms of diminished capacity to interpret environmental stimuli. At the same time, energy that is generated from conflicts as a result of person-environment interactions is lost (Riegel, 1979). In the final stage of the disease, afflicted persons also lose physical energy input from the environment because they cannot swallow nourishments. The outcome of this gradual process is loss of capacity to develop.

There is support for such theorizing. Prigogine, a physical chemist, won the 1977 Nobel Prize for his demonstration that both physical and biologic systems can be negentropic (can increase their levels of energy and organization) but only at the expense of the system's local environment (Prigogine, 1978). During early years of a person's development, the local surroundings become depleted of resources. People broaden their range of environmental interactions not only because of increased social skills but also for continued survival. Consequently, when the capacity to interact with the environment diminishes, survival is threatened and eventually development will cease. Interaction with the environment, therefore, becomes increasingly important for people's well-being as they age (Reed, 1983).

In Alzheimer's disease, the mind loses its capacity to interact with the environment and with people through significant gestures of shared meaning. The Alzheimer's afflicted mind increasingly loses the capacity for subjective experience and to observe its own actions. What is uniquely human is lost, and this happens long before the physical body loses its capacity for using energy from the environment. But, as Mead has pointed out, the body is not a self (or person with human capacities). A self exists only through a developed mind "within the context of social experience" (Mead, 1977, p. 161). An Alzheimer's disease afflicted person once had such a developed mind, but the illness evolves into The Loss of Self, to use Cohen and Eisdorfer's (1986) phrase. As the social process is lost, as interactions between person and environment cease, the self diminishes until, like the smile of Lewis Carroll's Cheshire cat, all that is left is an outer physical sign. The social self is lost, and with its passing, the possibility of further development also comes to an end.

Unfortunately this negative portrayal of human decline is, to date, the final outcome for Alzheimer's disease afflicted persons.

But there is hope. Intense biomedical research into the causes of Alzheimer's disease is in progress, and although a cure may not be known in the immediate future, a number of medications are being tested that enhance memory functioning and that could slow down the disease process. This delay means that interactions between afflicted persons and their caregivers can continue for longer time periods. Such interactions provide energy for afflicted persons. In addition, caregivers are being taught to become more successful in structuring interactions geared to the level of afflicted persons' ability. Thus, instead of pushing afflicted persons farther into social isolation, interactions are increased. The energy input that afflicted persons derive from the environment therefore is maintained or even enhanced.

As this study poignantly demonstrated, many early to middle stage afflicted spouses are aware of their spouses' feelings. When they sense rejection, afflicted spouses decrease interactions; when they feel abandoned, they demand interactions; and when they feel understood, they enjoy interactions. Caregivers have more power to influence outcomes than they may realize.

A FINAL NOTE

Many hours were expended in documenting the impact of Alzheimer's disease on the marital relationship. Some findings will be relevant to only a few couples; others are important issues for all who care for an Alzheimer's afflicted spouse. But all who come into contact with caregiver spouses and their afflicted mates will, it is hoped, have gained in awareness and understanding of the issues faced by these couples.

The most important implications for practice brought to light by this study can be summarized as follows:

1. Money management is one of the major responsibilities a caregiver spouse has to assume—even when there is only the suspicion of memory loss.
2. Some caregivers make intense efforts to keep feelings of tension under control, and this can adversely affect their health.

3. Some afflicted spouses are easy to live with; others show clinging and demanding behavior. Caregivers who have a high need for other companionship need assistance with making suitable arrangements; help from other family members may need to be mobilized.

4. Affection and sexuality remain important issues even in the presence of Alzheimer's disease. A small number of afflicted males can become highly sexually active; caregivers need help in dealing with such behavior and with finding a male respite worker.

5. The caregivers' commitment to the future of the relationship is strongly influenced by their own health; facilitating timely and appropriate health care for caregivers has to become a priority for health care workers.

In light of these findings, health care professionals should keep the following most basic assessment questions in mind when talking with caregiver spouses:

1. Who handles the family finances, and what long-term financial arrangements have you made?

2. What causes tension between you and your spouse, and how do you handle it?

3. What do you and your spouse do together, and do you have a need to get away?

4. How much affection and sexual intimacy is there between you and your spouse, and are there problems?

5. What are your plans for the future?

6. How depressed do you feel?

7. Do *you* have health problems, and do *you* get proper care?

Intervention guidelines have been described in the preceding chapters. Health care professionals have the responsibility to teach, convey factual information to caregivers, and to help them make decisions. But it is equally important to convey to caregivers that their own emotional and physical health must be maintained. Their health provides the energy for interacting with their afflicted spouses, and interactions make a difference.

Appendix

The information provided in this section is intended primarily for researchers and students. Methodological and analytic strategies will be described.

SAMPLE SELECTION

The sample was selected purposively through 10 agencies/ organizations located in two southeastern states. Couples were notified first by the agencies/organizations. Subsequently the researcher made a phone contact to those who had expressed an interest in participating in the study. A brief assessment of whether the couple met inclusion criteria was made over the phone—that is, (a) the couple had to be married and living together at home, and (b) the impaired spouse had to be able to perform some ADL activities, communicate verbally, and recognize the spouse by name. An interview time was arranged for those who met inclusion criteria; major holidays, the couple's wedding anniversary date, and the birthday of either spouse were omitted for scheduling. All subjects gave their own written consent at the time of the home visit.

In total, 72 couples were contacted; 12 refused to be interviewed, and 13 did not meet study criteria. The final sample consisted of 47 couples, 30 with caregiver-afflicted spouse dyads and 17 with both spouses relatively healthy.

PSYCHOMETRIC INFORMATION ON SCALES

The Dyadic Adjustment Rating Scale (Spanier, 1976; Spanier & Filsinger, 1983; Spanier & Thompson, 1982) is a widely used scale with established criterion-related validity ($p < .001$), construct validity ($p < .001$), and internal consistency reliability (alpha .96). The scale has four subscales that respectively measure consensus/instrumental issues, tension, cohesion/companionship, and affection/sexuality. Spanier and Thompson (1982), using a confirmatory factor analysis, found that the four subscale factors accounted for 94% of the covariance among the items and that three of the subscales were quite well replicated. However, the affection/sexuality subscale factor was found to be statistically orthogonal to the other three factors. The authors recommended that additional items measuring affectional expression be generated. This augmentation was accomplished with this study by adding five new items: touching the spouse lovingly, caressing the spouse, holding hands, putting an arm around the spouse, and sleeping in the same bed. The items were scored in the same manner as one of the original items (kissing the spouse). The new affection items yielded an alpha of .89. The combination of old and new affection items achieved an alpha of .88, and all affection and sex items combined achieved an alpha of .85.

Alphas for the other subscales were as follows: .88 for consensus/instrumental issues, .74 for tension, and .76 for cohesion/companionship. Chapters 2, 3, 4, and 5 present findings related to the four subscales.

It should be noted that the scoring used by Spanier and Thompson (1982) for individual scale items ranged from 0 to 6, or 0 to 5, or 0 to 1, yielding a maximum score of 151, based on 32 items. The scale adapted for this study had a constant of 1 added to each item to avoid zero scoring. Thus the maximum score on the revised scale (which included five new affection items) was 210.

Commitment to the Spouse was an additional marital quality measure. The two questions "Why did you marry?" and "Why have you stayed married?" were based on Swensen and Trahaug's (1985) differentiation of commitment in long-term marriages: Commitment can be based on viewing marriage as an institution or on valuing the spouse as a unique person. These two questions also provided a longitudinal assessment from the beginning of a couple's relationship to the present.

Swensen and Trahaug (1985) reported interjudge reliability for the answers as .83 and that answers differentiated between happily married couples (who valued the spouse as unique person) and unhappily married couples (who valued marriage as an institution).

Answers obtained from spouses in this study were given a random number and were copied onto work sheets. Four independent raters scored each answer on a continuum of 1 through 5, with 4 and 5 indicating that the spouse was valued as a unique person, 1 and 2 that marriage was valued as an institution, and 3 that the answer was equally strong in both sentiments; for example, "I love him. We made a lifetime commitment."

For the question "Why did you marry?" interrater reliability was .85. For the question "Why have you stayed married?" interrater reliability was .95. Findings pertaining to this measure are discussed in Chapter 6.

The Short Zung Interviewer Assisted Depression Rating Scale, referred to as the Short Zung I.D.S. (Tucker et al., 1986, 1987), is a 10-item scale particularly suitable for screening depression in older people. The scale has high correlations with the depression scale of the Minnesota Multiphasic Personality Inventory (r .70) and the Hamilton Depression Rating Scale (r. 41 to .56). A diagnosis of depression was confirmed on interview by psychiatrists using *DSM-III* criteria in elderly patients who obtained a depression score of greater than 70 on the Short Zung.

Subjects were asked to rate the following items based on feelings for the last 2 weeks or longer: feeling downhearted and blue, having trouble sleeping at night, feeling best in the morning (scoring reversed), eating as much as ever (scoring reversed), getting tired for no reason, finding it difficult to make decisions, feeling hopeful about the future (scoring reversed), feeling useful and needed (scoring reversed), feeling that life is somewhat empty, and still enjoying things as much as before (scoring reversed). Each item has a range of scoring from *seldom or never* (1) to *most of the time* (4). The total obtained score is divided by 40 and multiplied by 100, yielding a *Zung Index*. Interviewers should immediately check the answers given by respondents because, in this study, many spouses did not pay attention to positively versus negatively phrased items and would have given incorrect answers if not questioned about their scores.

Alpha for this sample was .75. In Chapter 6, only the caregivers' depression scores are discussed. None of the caregivers had a score of ≥70; their scores, therefore, should be considered an indication of dysphoric moods but not clinical depression.

The Multiple Assessment Instrument (MAI) developed by Lawton et al. (1982) and abbreviated by Weinberger et al. (1986) assesses several aspects of physical health. The scale correlates highly with other health ratings (.79) and has previously reported internal reliability (alpha) of .66. Scale items include self-rated health, ranging from *excellent* (4) to *poor* (1); whether health problems stop desired activities, ranging from *not at all* (4) to *completely* (1); whether a wheelchair is used, ranging from *never* (3) to *always* (1); number of doctor visits and days of hospitalization during the past year, ranging from *none* (4) to ≥8 (1) for doctor visits and ≥15 (1) for hospitalizations; number of medications taken per day, ranging from *none* (4) to ≥15/day (1); and absence or presence of heart and circulatory problems, ranging from *yes* (2) to *no* (1). A maximum score of 27 indicates perfect health, while a minimum score of 8 indicates very poor health. The internal reliability coefficient, alpha, for this sample was .76. In Chapter 6, only the caregivers' health scores are discussed. None of the caregivers in this study used a wheelchair.

The Jalowiec Coping Scale (Jalowiec, 1988; Jalowiec, Murphy, & Powers, 1984; Jalowiec & Powers, 1981) has well-documented content validity, test-retest reliability ($p < .0001$), internal consistency (alpha .86), and confirmatory factor analysis construct validity for the three subconstructs (subscales). For this sample, alpha for the total scale was .87. The subscales achieved alphas of .81 for confrontive coping, .78 for palliative coping, and .72 for emotive coping. The maximum score on the 40-item Jalowiec Coping Scale is 160, based on item scoring ranging from 0 to 4. In this study a constant of 1 was added to each item to avoid zero scoring. Thus the maximum obtainable score was 200. Findings based on the Jalowiec Coping Scale are discussed in Chapter 7.

QUALITATIVE DATA

The interview questionnaire contained several open-ended questions; in particular, coping with specific marital issues was explored with such questions as: "Do you have problems with . . . ?" "What type of problems?" "What do you do if . . . ?" "What else do you do . . . ?" "Who would help you?"

Answers to these open-ended questions were analyzed for emergent themes; categories and related categories were formed and cross tabulated to show interaction patterns (Glaser & Strauss, 1971; Stern, 1985). To establish trustworthiness of the qualitative data (Lincoln & Guba, 1985), attention was paid to negative cases, referring back to extensive observational notes, and, if clarification was needed, subjects were recontacted by phone. Triangulation of qualitative and quantitative data has been demonstrated throughout the book. Particularly noteworthy is Chapter 3, in which marital tension is discussed. Only through the combination of qualitative and quantitative data was the mind-set of caregivers brought into focus and could meaningful interpretation of low tension (deliberately kept low) be made.

VALIDITY AND RELIABILITY OF DATA OBTAINED FROM AFFLICTED SPOUSES

Very few studies with samples from the dementia population have attempted to include the perspective of the care *receiver*. The assumption seems to be that such information is invalid and unreliable for research purposes. As findings from this study indicate, however, afflicted spouses in the late confusional phase can provide a wealth of information, particularly if interviewed in their own environment and if a slow pace and cue cards as visual aids are used. Studies by Davis and Robins (1989) also indicate that those with a Mini-Mental State score of 18 or higher can answer questions quite accurately.

Distorted perceptions may indeed be exposed when afflicted spouses' answers are compared to those of their caregivers. But this comparison is valid information because it provides access to the lived experience of afflicted persons. To ignore their perceptions is arrogant behavior on the part of researchers. Researchers have the responsibility of ferreting out who is distorting facts—it could be the caregivers!

But reliability and validity issues are important when comparisons between AD group and well group couples are made. A special technique was developed to ensure valid comparisons of data obtained with quantitated scales; this technique is detailed below.

DATA ANALYSIS WITH QUANTITATED SCALES

Analysis of data obtained from quantitated scales focused on two major issues: (a) differences (or agreement) between husband and wife dyads and (b) differences between AD and well group couples.

Differences or agreement between husband and wife dyads is referred to as *within-couple comparison.* Two-factor analyses of variance (ANOVAs) with repeated measures and post hoc paired *t* tests were used to test the extent to which husbands and wives agreed or differed on specific issues. Although the robustness of ANOVA techniques is generally acknowledged even with small samples, nonparametric Wilcoxon Signed-Rank tests also were used; these yielded identical significance levels. Several instances of differences in perception between husbands and wives were exposed.

Differences between the AD and well group couples are referred to as *between-couple comparisons.* Two-factor ANOVAs and

Fisher's least significant difference (LSD) post hoc tests were used to analyze group differences that helped differentiate between illness impact and normal aging. Nonparametric Kruskal-Wallis analyses yielded identical significance levels. But when comparing AD and well group couples, concerns over validity and reliability of scores obtained from afflicted spouses had to be taken into consideration. Thus, for group comparisons, only the caregiver spouses' answers were used to represent the AD group, and for the well group, a random sample of 4 male and 13 female spouses (only one from each couple) was selected in order to be consistent with the 1:4 male/female caregiver ratio. Data contrasting between-couple and within-couple comparisons are detailed in Tables 2.1, 3.3, 4.1, 5.2, and 6.1.

Group comparisons for frequency of sexual contacts shown in Table 5.1 also use only the caregiver spouses' answers and those of 13 female and 4 male well group spouses, one per couple and randomly selected. Because husbands and wives from the well group gave practically identical answers regarding frequency of sexual contacts, a mean couple score yields identical results and could have been used for this analysis. However, the one-per-couple selection was chosen to keep all analyses consistent.

LIMITATIONS AND RECOMMENDATIONS FOR FUTURE RESEARCH

No study is complete without pointing to its limitations and to suggestions for further research. Both will be addressed.

Limitations

The marital relationships described in this book are based on interviews with 30 caregiver-afflicted couples and 17 relatively healthy couples. Although this totals 94 in-depth interviews, it is still a relatively small sample, which poses limitations for generalizing the information to the population of spouse caregivers.

In addition, more advanced statistical analyses cannot be performed with the present data. For example, Figure 1.1 shows relationships between important variables in this study. To test the entire model simultaneously requires a much larger sample. In addition to a larger sample, the use of quantitated and preferably standardized scales is necessary when testing a structural equation model or when performing other advanced statistical analyses. Although a number of standardized scales were used in this study, the theoretical constructs being measured by such scales was not entirely apparent when the instruments were selected. As this investigation has shown, no significant difference between groups on a quantitated marital tension scale does not mean there is no difference. The researcher had to question why certain answers were given. Additional qualitative data and triangulation methods led to more valid conclusions.

The measurement of coping with a quantitated scale also required careful evaluation. Coping is situation specific, and unless the investigator knows the mind-set of the people who answer the scale items, measurement of coping can be meaningless. Fortunately the standardized coping scale was just one aspect of the investigation. Answers to open-ended questions helped put the quantified information into its appropriate context.

Another potential limitation is the accuracy of responses obtained from afflicted spouses. Indeed, distorted perceptions were exposed on several occasions. Yet the intent was to gain access to afflicted persons' phenomenological world, and, as such, accuracy or reliability is not the major issue.

Recommendations for Future Research

In future studies a highly sensitive microphone and a high-quality recorder should be used. With appropriate equipment, recorded responses will be audible, particularly from afflicted spouses. Tapes can be transcribed, and researchers would not have to rely solely on the interviewer's speed of writing (although notes should still be taken). In addition, it is advisable to have two interviewers present during a home visit. This pairing would have several advantages: It will decrease the time required to obtain the desired information; caregiver spouses will be more relaxed, knowing that another person is there to watch the mate; and two interviewers can record interactions between spouses, thus providing a reliability check of observational data. The use of comparison groups is highly recommend and could be expanded to other illness situations. Only through comparisons can we begin to understand the relative impact of major developmental crises. In addition, a longitudinal perspective is required when studying development. Follow-up studies and replicated studies are necessary to determine intradevelopmental, versus cohort, versus historical issues (Botwinick, 1984).

Whether current levels of marital quality or caregiver health can predict institutionalization are intradevelopmental issues. On the other hand, commitment to the spouse can be a cohort issue. The couples in this study belonged to a generation with high commitment to traditional marriage vows. The present younger generations—who will be the older cohorts of tomorrow— may not view marriage as a lifelong commitment.

Historical issues involve the extent to which present versus future formal social support and health care programs influence the couples' lives. All of these issues are important considerations in future research. They are at the same time developmental issues in the broadest sense: Researchers and those who are the focus of investigations become transformed "from the outside in." But only when we lose the capacity to take cues and energy from the environment and when, in turn, we lose the capacity to influence our environment does development cease.

References

Anthony, J. C., LeResche, L., Niaz, U., von Korff, M. R., & Folstein, M. F. (1982). Limits of the "Mini-Mental State" as a screening test for dementia and delirium among hospital patients. *Psychological Medicine, 12,* 397-408.

Antonovsky, A. (1987). *Unravelling the mystery of health.* San Francisco: Jossey-Bass.

Baldwin, B. A. (1988). Community management of Alzheimer's disease. *Nursing Clinics of North America, 23,* 47-56.

Baldwin, B. A. (1990). Family caregiving: Trends and forecasts. *Geriatric Nursing, 11,* 172-174.

Baltes, P. B. (1979). Life-span developmental psychology: Some converging observations on history and theory. In P. B. Baltes & O. G. Brim, Jr. (Eds.), *Life-span development and behavior* (pp. 256-281). New York: Academic Press.

Barusch, A. S. (1988). Problems and coping strategies of elderly spouse caregivers. *The Gerontologist, 28,* 677-685.

Beck, C., & Heacock, P. (1988). Nursing interventions for patients with Alzheimer's disease. *Nursing Clinics of North America, 23,* 95-124.

Beck, C., Heacock, P., Mercer, S., Walton, C. G., & Shook, J. (1991). Dressing for success. Promoting independence among cognitively impaired elderly. *Journal of Psychosocial Nursing, 29,* 30-35.

Beck, C. M., & Phillips, L. R. (1983). Abuse of the elderly. *Journal of Gerontological Nursing, 9,* 97-101.

Beisecker, A. E., Wright, L., & Kasal, S. (1991). *Medical encounters involving physicians, family caregivers, and patients with Alzheimer's disease.* (Paper presented at the 44th Annual Scientific Meeting of the Gerontological Society of America). *The Gerontologist, 31,* 154.

Bergman, K., & Cooper, B. (1986). Epidemiological and public health aspects of senile dementia. In A. B. Soerensen, F. E. Weiner, & L. R. Sherwoods (Eds.), *Human development and the life course: Multidisciplinary perspectives* (pp. 71-97). Hillsdale, NJ: Lawrence Erlbaum.

Botwinick, J. (1984). *Aging and behavior.* New York: Springer.

Brandtstaedter, J. (1984). Person and social control over development: Some implications of an action perspective in life-span developmental psychology. In P. B. Baltes & O. G. Brim, Jr. (Eds.), *Life-span development and behavior* (Vol. 6, pp. 1-32). New York: Academic Press.

Brubaker, T. H. (1985). *Later life families.* Beverly Hills, CA: Sage.

Burns, E. M., & Buckwalter, K. C. (1988). Pathophysiology of Alzheimer's disease. *Nursing Clinics of North America, 23,* 11-29.

Cantor, M. H. (1983). Strain among caregivers: A study of experience in the United States. *The Gerontologist, 23,* 597-604.

Caserta, M. S., Lund, D. A., Wright, S. D., & Redburn, D. E. (1987). Caregivers to dementia patients: The utilization of community services. *The Gerontologist, 27,* 209-214.

Chappell, N. L., & Badger, M. (1989). Social isolation and well-being. *Journal of Gerontology, 44,* S169-176.

Chappell, N. L., & Orbach, H. L. (1986). Socialization in old age: A Meadian perspective. In V. W. Marshall (Ed.), *Later life* (pp. 75-106). Beverly Hills, CA: Sage.

Clipp, E. C., & George, L. K. (1990). Caregiver needs and patterns of social support. *Journal of Gerontology, 45,* S102-111.

Cohen, D., & Eisdorfer, C. (1986). *The loss of self.* New York: Penguin.

Colerick, E., & George, L. K. (1986). Predictors of institutionalization among caregivers of patients with Alzheimer's disease. *Journal of the American Geriatrics Society, 34,* 493-498.

Coser, L. A. (1977). *Masters of sociological thought.* Orlando, FL: Harcourt Brace Jovanovich.

Cutrona, C. E., & Russell, D. W. (1987). Provisions of social relationships and adaptation to stress. *Advances in Personal Relationships, 1,* 37-67.

Davis, B. A. (1985). Commentary to "Adjustment patterns of chronically ill middle-aged persons and spouses" by M. J. Foxall, J. Y. Ekberg, and N. Griffith. *Western Journal of Nursing Research, 7,* 425-444.

Davis, P. B., & Robins, L. N. (1989). History-taking in the elderly with and without cognitive impairment. *Journal of the American Geriatrics Society, 37,* 249-255.

Deimling, G. T., & Poulshock, S. W. (1985). The transition from family in-home care to institutional care. *Research on Aging, 7,* 563-576.

Dowd, J. J. (1990). Ever since Durkheim: The socialization of human development. *Human Development, 33,* 138-159.

Dura, J. R., Haywood-Niler, E., & Kiecolt-Glaser, J. K. (1990). Spousal caregivers of persons with Alzheimer's and Parkinson's disease dementia: A preliminary comparison. *The Gerontologist, 30,* 332-336.

Eisdorfer, C. (1991). Caregiving: An emerging risk factor for emotional and physical pathology. *Bulletin of the Menninger Clinic, 55,* 238-247.

Emmons, C. A., Biernat, M., Tiedje, L. B., Lang, E. L., & Wortman, C. B. (1990). Stress, support, and coping among women professionals with preschool children. In J. Eckenroade & S. Gore (Eds.), *Stress between work and family* (pp. 61-93). New York: Plenum.

Enright, R. B. (1991). Time spent caregiving and help received by spouses and adult children of brain-impaired adults. *The Gerontologist, 31,* 375-383.

Evans, D. A., Funkenstein, H. H., Albert, M. S., Scherr, P. A., Cook, N. R., Chown, M. J., Herbert, L. E., Hennekens, C. H., & Taylor, J. O. (1989). Prevalence of Alzheimer's disease in a community population of older persons: Higher than previously reported. *Journal of the American Medical Association, 252,* 2551-2556.

Farran, C. J., & Keane-Hagerty, E. (1989). Communicating effectively with dementia patients. *Journal of Psychosocial Nursing, 27,* 13-16.

Feldman, S. S., Biringen, Z. C., & Nash, S. C. (1981). Fluctuations of sex-related self-attributions as a function of stage of family cycle. *Developmental Psychology, 17,* 24-35.

Ferris, S. H., deLeon, M. J., Wolf, A. P., et al. (1980). Positron tomography in the study of aging and senile dementia. *Neurobiology of Aging, 1,* 127-131.

Folkman, S., & Lazarus, R. S. (1980). An analysis of coping in a middle-aged community sample. *Journal of Health and Social Behavior, 21,* 219-239.

Folstein, M. F., Folstein, S. E., & McHugh, P. R. (1975). Mini-Mental State. *Journal of Psychiatric Research, 12,* 189-198.

Garrison, H., & Howe, A. (1976). Community intervention with the elderly: A social network approach. *Journal of the American Geriatrics Society, 24,* 329-333.

George, L., Fillenbaum, G., & Burchett, B. (1988). *Respite care: A strategy for easing caregiver burden.* Durham, NC: Duke University Medical Center, Center for the Study of Aging and Human Development.

George, L. K., & Gwyther, L. P. (1986). Caregiver well-being: A multidimensional examination of family caregivers of demented adults. *The Gerontologist, 26,* 253-259.

Georgoudi, M. (1983). Modern dialectics in social psychology: A reappraisal. *European Journal of Social Psychology, 13,* 1-17.

Gilford, R. (1984). Contrasts in marital satisfaction throughout old age: An exchange theory analysis. *Journal of Gerontology, 39,* 325-333.

Gilleard, C. J., Gilleard, E., Gledhill, K., & Whittick, J. (1984). Caring for the elderly mentally infirm at home: A survey of the supporters. *Journal of Epidemiology and Community Health, 38,* 319-325.

Given, C. W., Collins, C. E., & Given, B. A. (1988). Sources of stress among families caring for relatives with Alzheimer's disease. *Nursing Clinics of North America, 23,* 69-82.

Glaser, B. G., & Strauss, A. L. (1971). *The discovery of grounded theory.* Hawthorne, NY: Aldine.

Gove, W. R., Hughes, M., & Style, B. C. (1983). Does marriage have positive effects on psychological well-being of the individual? *Journal of Health and Social Behavior, 24,* 122-131.

Green, V. L., & Monahan, D. J. (1987). The effect of professionally guided caregiver support and education groups on institutionalization of care receivers. *The Gerontologist, 27,* 716-721.

Gwyther, L. P. (1988). Nursing-home care issues. In M. K. Aronson (Ed.), *Understanding Alzheimer's disease* (pp. 238-262). New York: Scribner.

Gwyther, L. P., & Matteson, M. A. (1983). Care for the caregivers. *Journal of Gerontological Nursing, 9,* 92-95, 110, 116.

Haan, N. (1977). *Coping and defending.* New York: Academic Press.

Haley, W. E., Levine, E. G., Brown, S. L., & Barolucci, A. A. (1987). Stress, appraisal, coping, and social support as predictors of adaptational outcome among dementia caregivers. *Psychology and Aging, 2,* 323-330.

Hall, G. R. (1988). Care of the patient with Alzheimer's disease living at home. *Nursing Clinics of North America, 23,* 31-46.

Hamel, M., Gold, D. P., Andres, D., Reis, M., Dastoor, D., Grauer, H., & Bergman, H. (1990). Predictors and consequences of aggressive behavior by community-based dementia patients. *The Gerontologist, 30,* 206-211.

Harvis, K. A. (1990). Care plan approach to dementia. *Geriatric Nursing, 11,* 76-80.

Heacock, P., Walton, C., Beck, C., & Mercer, S. (1991). Caring for the cognitively impaired. Reconceptualizing disability and rehabilitation. *Journal of Gerontological Nursing, 17,* 22-26.

Hertz, R. (1986). *More equal than others.* Los Angeles: University of California Press.

Holahan, C. K. (1984). Marital attitudes over 40 years: A longitudinal and cohort analysis. *Journal of Gerontology, 39,* 49-57.

Jalowiec, A. (1988). Confirmatory factor analysis of the Jalowiec Coping Scale. In C. F. Waltz & O. L. Strickland (Eds.), *Measurement of nursing outcomes* (pp. 287-308). New York: Springer.

Jalowiec, A., Murphy, S. P., & Powers, M. J. (1984). Psychometric assessment of the Jalowiec Coping Scale. *Nursing Research, 33,* 157-161.

Jalowiec, A., & Powers, M. J. (1981). Stress and coping in hypertensive and emergency room patients. *Nursing Research, 30,* 10-15.

Joachim, C. L., & Selkoe, D. J. (1989). Minireview: Amyloid protein in Alzheimer's disease. *Journal of Gerontology, 44,* B77-82.

Kapust, L. R. (1982). Living with dementia: The ongoing funeral. *Social Work in Health Care, 7,* 79-91.

Lawton, M., Brody, E., & Saperstein, A. (1989). Respite care for Alzheimer's families: Research findings and their relevance to providers. *American Journal of Alzheimer's and Related Disorders Care and Research, 4,* 31-38.

Lawton, M. P., Moss, M., Fulcomer, M., & Kleban, M. H. (1982). A research and service-oriented multilevel assessment instrument. *Journal of Gerontology, 37,* 91-99.

Lazarus, R. S., Averill, J. R., & Opton, E. M., Jr. (1974). The psychology of coping: Issues of research assessment. In G. V. Coelho, D. A. Hamburg, & J. E. Adams (Eds.), *Coping and adaptation* (pp. 189-217). New York: Basic Books.

Lehr, U. M. (1982). Depression and "Lebensqualitaet" im Alter—Korrelate negativer und positiver Gestimmtheit. *Gerontologie, 15,* 241-249.

Lerner, R. M. (1985). Individual and context in developmental psychology: Conceptual and theoretical issues. In J. R. Nesselroad & A. von Eye (Eds.), *Individual development and social change* (pp. 155-187). New York: Academic Press.

Lerner, R. M., & Kauffman, M. B. (1985). The concept of development in contextualism. *Developmental Review, 5,* 309-333.

Liang, J. (1986). Self-reported physical health among aged adults. *Journal of Gerontology, 41,* 248-260.

Lieberman, M. A., & Kramer, J. H. (1991). Factors affecting decisions to institutionalize demented elderly. *The Gerontologist, 31,* 371-374.

Lieberman, M. A., & Tobin, S. S. (1983). *The experience of old age: Stress, coping, and survival.* New York: Basic Books.

Lincoln, Y. S., & Guba, E. G. (1985). *Naturalistic inquiry.* Beverly Hills, CA: Sage.

Lindgren, C. L. (1990). Burnout and social support in family caregivers. *Western Journal of Nursing Research, 12,* 469-487.

Litz, B. T., Zeiss, A. M., & Davies, H. D. (1990). Sexual concerns of male spouses of female Alzheimer's disease patients. *The Gerontologist, 30,* 113-116.

Longino, C., & Lipman, A. (1981). Married and spouseless men and women in planned retirement communities: Support network differentials. *Journal of Marriage and the Family, 43,* 169-177.

Lund, D. A., Pett, M. A., & Caserta, M. S. (1987). Institutionalizing dementia victims: Some caregiver considerations. *Journal of Gerontological Social Work, 11,* 119-135.

Maas, M., Buckwalter, K., & Kelley, L. (1991a). Characteristics and perceptions of care of family members of institutionalized patients with Alzheimer's disease: A brief report. *Applied Nursing Research, 4,* 135-140.

Maas, M., Buckwalter, K., & Kelley, L. (1991b). Family members' perceptions: How they view care of Alzheimer's patients in a nursing home. *Journal of Long Term Care Administration, 19,* 21-25.

Macken, C. L. (1986). A profile of functionally impaired elderly persons living in the community. *Health Care Financing Review, 7,* 33-49.

Magaziner, J., Bassett, S. P., & Hebel, J. R. (1987). Predicting performance on the Mini-Mental State examination. Use of age- and education-specific equations. *Journal of the American Geriatrics Society, 35,* 996-1000.

McCubbin, H. I., Cauble, A. E., & Patterson, J. M. (1982). *Family stress, coping, and social support.* Springfield, IL: Charles C Thomas.

McCulloch, A. W. (1981). What do we mean by "development" in old age? *Aging and Society, 1,* 229-245.

McFall, S., & Miller, B. H. (1990). The impact of caregiver burden on nursing home admission by frail elderly. *The Gerontologist, 30,* 168A.

Mead, G. H. (1934). *Mind, self, and society.* Chicago: University of Chicago Press.

Mead, G. H. (1977). *On social psychology.* Chicago: University of Chicago Press.

Menninger, K. (1963). *The vital balance: The process in mental health and illness.* New York: Viking.

Miller, B. (1987). Gender and control among spouses of the cognitively impaired: A research note. *The Gerontologist, 27,* 447-453.

Mitchell, L. (1991). *Medicare made easy. A practical guide.* Denver, CO: GeriMed of America.

Monga, T. N., Monga, M., Raina, M. S., & Hardjasudarma, M. (1986). Hypersexuality in stroke. *Archives of Physical Medicine and Rehabilitation, 67,* 415-417.

Montgomery, R., & Borgatta, E. (1989). The effects of alternative support strategies on family caregiving. *The Gerontologist, 29,* 457-464.

Moos, R. H. (1977). *Coping with physical illness.* New York: Plenum.

Neugarten, B. L., & Gutmann, D. L. (1958). Age-sex roles and personality in middle age: A thematic apperception study [Whole issue]. *Psychological Monographs: General and Applied, 17,*(470).

Noelker, L., & Kercher, K. (1991). Perceived burden and well-being of elderly receiving family care. (Paper presented at the 44th Annual Scientific Meeting of the Gerontological Society of America). *The Gerontologist, 31,* 52.

Office of Technology Assessment (OTA). (1987). *Losing a million minds* (OTA-BA-323). Washington, DC: Government Printing Office.

Office of Technology Assessment (OTA). (1990). *Confused minds, burdened families* (OTA-BA-403). Washington, DC: Government Printing Office.

Overman, W., Jr., & Stoudemire, A. (1988). Guidelines for legal and financial counseling of Alzheimer's disease patients and their families. *American Journal of Psychiatry, 145,* 1495-1500.

Pearlin, L. I., Mullan, J. T., Semple, S. J., & Skaff, M. M. (1990). Caregiving and the stress process: An overview of concepts and their measures. *The Gerontologist, 30,* 583-594.

Pearlin, L. I., & Schooler, C. (1978). The structure of coping. *Journal of Health and Social Behavior, 19,* 2-21.

Prigogine, I. (1978). Time, structure, and fluctuation. *Science, 201,* 777-785.

Pruchno, R. A. (1990). The effects of help patterns on the mental health of spouse caregivers. *Research on Aging, 12,* 57-71.

Pruchno, R. A., Michaels, J. E., & Potashnik, S. L. (1990). Predictors of institutionalization among Alzheimer's disease victims with caregiving spouses. *Journal of Gerontology, 45,* S259-266.

Quayhagen, M. P., & Quayhagen, M. (1988). Alzheimer's stress: Coping with the caregiving role. *The Gerontologist, 28,* 391-396.

Ray, C., Lindop, J., & Gibson, S. (1982). The concept of coping. *Psychological Medicine, 12,* 385-395.

Reed, P. G. (1983). Implications of the life-span developmental framework for well-being in adulthood and aging. *Advances in Nursing Science, 6,* 18-25.

Reedy, M. N., Birren, M. E., & Schaie, K. W. (1982). Age and sex differences in satisfying love relationships across the adult life span. In K. W. Schaie & J. Geiwitz (Eds.), *Readings in adult development and aging* (pp. 154-165). Boston: Little, Brown.

Reisberg, B. (1983). Clinical presentation, diagnosis, and symptomatology of age associated cognitive decline and Alzheimer's disease. In B. Reisberg (Ed.), *Alzheimer's disease: The standard reference* (pp. 173-187). New York: Free Press.

Riegel, K. F. (1973). Dialectical operations: The final period of cognitive development. *Human Development, 16,* 346-470.

Riegel, K. F. (1976). The dialects of human development. *American Psychologist, 31,* 689-700.

Riegel, K. F. (1979). *Foundations of dialectical psychology.* New York: Academic Press.

Roberts, B. L., & Algase, D. L. (1988). Victims of Alzheimer's disease and the environment. *Nursing Clinics of North America, 23,* 83-93.

Robinson, K. (1988). Older women who are caregivers. *Health Care for Women International, 9,* 239-249.

Robinson, K. M. (1989). Predictors of depression among wife caregivers. *Nursing Research, 38,* 359-363.

Robinson, K. M. (1990a). Predictors of burden among wife caregivers. *Scholarly Inquiry for Nursing Practice: An International Journal, 4,* 189-203.

Robinson, K. M. (1990b). The relationship between social skills, social support, self-esteem, and burden in adult caregivers. *Journal of Advanced Nursing, 15,* 788-795.

Rothenthal, C. J., & Dawson, P. (1991). Wives of institutionalized men. *Journal of Aging and Health, 3,* 315-334.

Ryff, C. D. (1984). Personality development from the inside: The subjective experience of change in adulthood and aging. In P. B. Baltes & O. G. Brim (Eds.), *Life-span development and behavior* (pp. 243-279). New York: Academic Press.

Schulz, R., Visantainer, P., & Williamson, G. M. (1990). Psychiatric and physical morbidity effects of caregiving. *Journal of Gerontology, 45,* P181-191.

Shanas, E. (1979). Social myth as hypothesis: The case of the family relations of old people. *The Gerontologist, 19,* 3-9.

Silliman, R. A., & Sternberg, J. (1988). Family caregiving: Impact of patient functioning and underlying causes of dependency. *The Gerontologist, 28,* 377-382.

Simmel, G. (1950). *The sociology of Georg Simmel* (K. H. Wolff, Ed. and Trans.). New York: Free Press.

Sjogren, T., Sjogren, H., & Lundgren, G. H. (1952). Clinical analysis of morbus Alzheimer and morbus Pick. *Acta Psychiatrica Scandanavia* (Supp. 82), 69-115.

Snyder, B., & Keefe, K. (1985). The unmet needs of family caregivers for frail and disabled adults. *Social Work in Health Care, 10,* 1-14.

Snyder, L. H., Rupprecht, P., Pyret, J., Brekhus, S., & Moss, T. (1978). Wandering. *The Gerontologist, 18,* 272-280.

Soldo, B. J., & Myllyluoma, J. (1983). Caregivers who live with dependent elderly. *The Gerontologist, 23,* 605-611.

Spanier, G. B. (1976). Measuring dyadic adjustment: New scales for assessing the quality of marriage and similar dyads. *Journal of Marriage and the Family, 32,* 15-28.

Spanier, G. B., & Filsinger, E. E. (1983). The dyadic adjustment scale. In E. E. Filsinger (Ed.), *Marriage and family assessment* (pp. 155-160). Beverly Hills, CA: Sage.

Spanier, G. B., Lewis, R. A., & Cole, C. L. (1975). Marital adjustment over the family life cycle: The issue of curvilinearity. *Journal of Marriage and the Family, 31,* 263-268.

Spanier, G. B., & Thompson, L. (1982). A confirmatory analysis of the dyadic adjustment scale. *Journal of Marriage and the Family, 38,* 731-741.

Special Committee on Aging. United States Senate. (1990). *Understanding Medicare: A guide for children of aging parents* (Serial No. 101-0). Washington, DC: Government Printing Office.

Starr, B. D. (1985). Sexuality and aging. *Annual Review of Gerontology and Geriatrics, 5,* 97-126.

Stern, P. N. (1985). Using grounded theory method in nursing research. In M. M. Leininger (Ed.), *Qualitative research methods in nursing* (pp. 149-160). New York: Grune & Stratton.

Stone, R., Cafferata, G. L., & Sangle, J. (1987). Caregivers of the frail elderly: A national profile. *The Gerontologist, 27,* 616-626.

Strain, L. A., & Chappell, N. L. (1982). Confidants. *Research on Aging, 4,* 479-502.

Swensen, C. H., & Trahaug, G. (1985). Commitment and the long-term marriage relationship. *Journal of Marriage and the Family, 41,* 939-945.

Thomas, W. I. (1923). *The unadjusted girl.* Boston: Little, Brown.

Tilden, V. P., & Galyen, R. D. (1987). Cost and conflict. The darker side of social support. *Western Journal of Nursing Research, 9*, 9-18.

Tucker, M. A., Ogle, S. J., Davinson, J. G., & Eilenberg, M. D. (1986). Development of a brief screening test for depression in the elderly. *Journal of Clinical and Experimental Gerontology, 8*, 173-190.

Tucker, M. A., Ogle, S. J., Davinson, J. G., & Eilenberg, M. D. (1987). Validation of a brief screening test for depression in the elderly. *Age and Ageing, 16*, 139-144.

Walz, T. H., & Blum, N. S. (1987). *Sexual health in later life.* Lexington, MA: D. C. Heath.

Weinberger, M., Darnell, J. C., Martz, B. L., Hiner, S. L., Neill, P. C., & Tierney, W. M. (1986). The effects of positive and negative life changes on the self-reported health status of elderly adults. *Journal of Gerontology, 41*, 114-119.

Weishaus, S., & Field, D. (1988). A half century of marriage: Continuity or change? *Journal of Marriage and the Family, 50*, 763-774.

Wright, L. K. (1989). Alzheimer's disease as developmental asynchrony: A dialectical paradigm of the marital relationship of older couples (Doctoral dissertation, University of Georgia, 1988). *Disertation Abstracts International, 49/11A*, 3518.

Wright, L. K. (1991a). The impact of Alzheimer's disease on the marital relationship. *The Gerontologist, 31*, 224-237.

Wright, L. K. (1991b). Predictors of in-home care for Alzheimer's disease afflicted spouses. *The Gerontologist, 31*, II, 154-155.

Yesavage, J. A., Brink, T. L., Rose, T. L., Lum, O., Huang, V., Adey, M., & von Leirer, O. (1983). Development and validation of a geriatric depression-screening scale: A preliminary report. *Journal of Psychiatric Research, 17*, 37-49.

Zarit, S. H., Reever, K. E., & Bach-Peterson, J. (1980). Relatives of the impaired elderly: Correlates of feelings of burden. *The Gerontologist, 20*, 649-655.

Zarit, S. H., Todd, P. A., & Zarit, J. M. (1986). Subjective burden of husbands and wives as caregivers: A longitudinal study. *The Gerontologist, 26*, 260-266.

Index

Abandonment fears, 69
Abuse, 42, 45. *See also* Verbal abuse
Acceptance stage, 67
Activities, joint, 56-57
Adaptation, 65, 67
Affect, flattening of, 4
Affection, 73-96, 122
    agreement over, 76
    amounts of, 74
    assessment strategies and, 94-95
    childlike, 77, 91
    human development and, 92-94
    intervention guidelines, 95-96
Afflicted couples:
    affection and, 74, 77-83, 85-91
    asynchronized life dimensions and,
        65
    awareness of spouse's feelings, 32-
        33, 121
    characteristics of, 11-12
    commitment and, 100-101, 105
    companionship and, 47-55
    future of relationship and, 101
    household tasks and, 24
    marital tension and, 32, 36-38, 39-40
    money management and, 21-22, 25-
        26
    relationship characteristics and, 112
    relationship patterns, 85-91

sexuality and, 77-83, 85-94
shared activities and, 47
Afflicted spouses:
    awareness of other and, 32-33, 121
    commitment and, 100, 105
    constricted life dimensions of, 66
    data received from, 127-128
    denial of problems, 40-41
    household tasks and, 15
    isolation of, 66
    marital tension and, 35, 36-38
    money management and, 21-22
    perspective of, 2
    sexual intimacy and, 74-76, 96
    social support and, 60, 61
    See also Female afflicted spouses;
        Male afflicted spouses
Agenda behavior, 43
Aging, problems associated with, 2
Aging trends, 6
Agitation, 42, 43
Aloneness, 51, 118
Alzheimer, Alois, 3
Alzheimer's disease:
    biological aspects of, 3
    biomedical research and, 121
    clinical aspects of, 4-5
    prevalence rate, 5
    sexual intimacy and, 74

About the Author

Lore K. Wright, PhD, RN, CS, recently completed a Postdoctoral Research Fellowship at the Center for Aging, Duke University Medical Center, Durham, North Carolina. She is now a faculty member at the Medical University of South Carolina in Charleston with joint appointments in the College of Medicine, Department of Psychiatry and Social Sciences, and the College of Nursing. Her nursing career spans clinical, administrative, teaching, and research positions. She has published in peer-reviewed journals such as *The Gerontologist, Journal of Psychosocial Nursing, Issues in Mental Health Nursing,* and *Journal of Nursing Administration.* Her research has been funded from both public and private funds. In 1989 she received the American Nurses' Association, Council of Nurse Researchers, prestigious Outstanding New Investigator Award for her research on the impact of Alzheimer's disease on the marital relationship.